Physical Activity Interventions in Children and Adolescents

Dianne S. Ward
University of North Carolina at Chapel Hill

Ruth P. Saunders
Russell R. Pate
University of South Carolina at Columbia

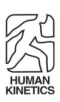

**HUMAN
KINETICS**

Library of Congress Cataloging-in-Publication Data

Ward, Dianne Stanton.
    Physical activity interventions in children and adolescents / Dianne S. Ward, Ruth P. Saunders, Russell R. Pate.
        p. cm.
    Includes bibliographical references and index.
    ISBN-13: 978-0-7360-5132-3 (soft cover)
    ISBN-10: 0-7360-5132-5 (soft cover)
    1. Physical fitness for children.   I. Saunders, Ruthie P.   II. Pate, Russell R.   III. Title.
    RJ133.W37 2007
    613.7'042--dc22

                                                            2006020608

ISBN-10: 0-7360-5132-5
ISBN-13: 978-0-7360-5132-3

Copyright © 2007 by Dianne S. Ward, Ruth P. Saunders, and Russell R. Pate

Permission notices for material reprinted in this book from other sources can be found on page xiii.

The Web addresses cited in this text were current as of July 2006, unless otherwise noted.

Acquisitions Editor: Michael S. Bahrke, PhD; **Developmental Editor:** Renee Thomas Pyrtel; **Assistant Editor:** Jillian Evans; **Copyeditor:** Joyce Sexton; **Proofreader:** John Wentworth; **Indexer:** Sharon Duffy; **Permission Manager:** Carly Breeding; **Graphic Designer:** Nancy Rasmus; **Graphic Artist:** Kathleen Boudreau-Fuoss; **Photo Manager:** Laura Fitch; **Cover Designer:** Keith Blomberg; **Photographer (cover):** Veer, Inc.; **Photographer (interior):** © Human Kinetics unless otherwise noted; **Art Manager:** Kelly Hendren; **Illustrator:** Denise Lowry; **Printer:** Versa Press

Printed in the United States of America   10 9 8 7 6 5 4 3 2

The paper in this book is certified under a sustainable forestry program.

Human Kinetics
Web site: www.HumanKinetics.com

United States: Human Kinetics
P.O. Box 5076
Champaign, IL 61825-5076
800-747-4457
e-mail: humank@hkusa.com

Canada: Human Kinetics
475 Devonshire Road, Unit 100
Windsor, ON N8Y 2L5
800-465-7301 (in Canada only)
e-mail: info@hkcanada.com

Europe: Human Kinetics
107 Bradford Road
Stanningley
Leeds LS28 6AT, United Kingdom
+44 (0)113 255 5665
e-mail: hk@hkeurope.com

Australia: Human Kinetics
57A Price Avenue
Lower Mitcham, South Australia 5062
08 8372 0999
e-mail: info@hkaustralia.com

New Zealand: Human Kinetics
P.O. Box 80
Torrens Park, South Australia 5062
0800 222 062
e-mail: info@hknewzealand.com

*We dedicate this book to the professionals
who work to help youth experience the joy
and reap the benefit of an active life
and to the children and young people
who make their—and our—efforts worthwhile.*

PART ONE   Physical Activity Behavior

PART TWO   Documented Interventions

The purpose of the Physical Activity Intervention Series is to publish texts, written by the leading researchers in the field, that provide specific and evidence-based methods and techniques for physical activity interventions. These books include practical suggestions, examples, forms, questionnaires, and specific intervention techniques that can be applied in field settings.

Many health professionals who currently provide exercise advice and offer exercise programs use the traditional and structured frequency, intensity, and time (FIT) approach to exercise prescription. Although the exercise prescription is valid, going to a fitness facility and participating in such programs are not attractive to many people, and there is a need to offer alternative programs based on the new consensus recommendations and using behavioral intervention methods and techniques.

The books in the Physical Activity Intervention Series provide information, methods, techniques, and support to the many health professionals—clinical exercise physiologists, nutritionists, physicians, fitness center exercise leaders, public health workers, and health promotion experts—who are looking for alternative ways to promote physical activity that do not require a rigid application of the FIT approach. It is to meet this need that Human Kinetics developed this Physical Activity Intervention Series.

The series has a broad scope. It includes books focused on after-school programs for children and youth, ways to implement physical activity interventions in the public health setting, and ways to evaluate physical activity interventions. The series also includes books that focus on the implementation of interventions based on theories and on interventions for other special populations such as older adults and those with chronic disease. Each book is valuable and useful in its own right, but the series will provide an integrated collection of materials that can be used to plan, develop, implement, and evaluate physical activity interventions in a wide variety of settings for diverse populations.

Physical activity is a cornerstone in the development of toddlers, young and older children, and adolescents approaching adulthood. However, today's way of life favors sedentary pursuits through the advancement of technology and innovation. We lead lives of convenience and enjoy passive entertainment with abundant availability of automobiles, computers, TVs and videos, electronic games, and labor-saving devices. Parents and educators worry about children's level of academic preparation for the 21st century and have responded by deprioritizing physical education while elevating class work and homework to the highest priority. Financial constraints in communities require that they choose between adding sidewalks and providing garbage service. In many two-parent families and in most single-parent ones, children's after-school time is in the hands of others or spent at home behind locked doors.

The downside of a modern life full of computers, cell phones, and automobiles is that today's youth can chat with friends or go to the mall without being physically active. Lack of engagement in active pursuits eliminates valuable opportunities for youth to enjoy physical stimulation and social–emotional development. The short-term health impact of a sedentary life is low energy expenditure and a risk of developing obesity. The long-term effect of youthful inactivity is increased risk of obesity, inadequate motor skill development, lack of competence to engage in sport or exercise, and an overall risk for a lower quality of life. In addition to these factors that are immediately relevant for youth, inactivity in youth leads to inactivity in adulthood, carrying with it the risk of cardiovascular disease, diabetes, high blood pressure, certain cancers, and even premature death.

This book has been written as a resource for professionals in schools, school districts, health departments, recreation centers, state agencies, and nonprofit organizations interested in developing programs to promote physical activity in children and adolescents. Because physical activity is very important to young people for optimal physical development and health, programs (sometimes called interventions) have been designed to increase regular physical activity participation, decrease sedentary behavior, or in some cases do both. Intervention is the term used to refer to a program designed to alter, or intervene on, a targeted behavior. For the purpose of this book, that behavior is physical activity.

Most documented interventions have been developed by university researchers and designed for home, school, or community settings. This book has been written to assist professionals who are interested in designing their own intervention or in using previously tested interventions with their local populations. For instance, a health educator from a local health department may want to find a physical activity program for use in public housing or with a local Girls & Boys Club, or a state or district physical education coordinator may want to find ways to increase physical activity levels of students during the school day. In addition, this book could be assigned as an ancillary textbook in a college curriculum for exercise science, health education, or physical education majors.

The book is partitioned into three sections. In chapters 1 through 3, we provide an orientation to activity in young people, describe how to change behavior, and introduce the settings in which such behavior change programs might be developed. This book also provides information on documented interventions that have been designed for a variety of settings: Chapter 4 deals with school settings, chapter 5 with the community, and chapter 6 with the family and physician. The last four chapters (7-10) have been developed to assist those who want to design their own intervention for a specific population or who wish to adapt existing interventions for the population with which they are working. These chapters can also be used to aid understanding of elements of existing interventions for better adaptation at the local level.

It is our hope that through the information provided, professionals can learn about physical activity and the role it plays in the lives of youth, how and where programs to change existing activity behavior could take place, and elements of building a successful program designed for one's own situation. We have provided examples of successful programs in a variety of settings and have presented tools for the development of new programs. Through this varied approach, it is our hope that you can successfully design, implement, and evaluate a program for physical activity.

The authors wish to thank the following individuals who contributed to the development of this book:

Kristina Killgrove, MA, who provided outstanding expertise in text and copyediting, and for her invaluable help in chasing down the final details of the authors' draft.

Richard Lawhon, PhD, who provided guidance and editorial skill in the formation of all chapters.

Amber Vaughn, MPH, for her background research in development of the intervention chapters.

Gaye Groover Christmus, MPH, for her skillful contributions to several sections of the book.

ACKNOWLEDGMENTS

Photos

Chapters 1, 5, 6, 7, 10 opener photos: © Margaret Holmes

Chapter 8 opener photo: © Bob Bergstrom Photography

Figure 8.1: Photo courtesy of ActiGraph, LLC.

Figure 8.4: © Photodisc

Tables

Table 2.1: Adapted from E.J. Stone, T.L. McKenzie, G.J. Welk and M.L. Booth, 1998, "Effects of physical activity interventions in youth: Review and synthesis," *American Journal of Preventive Medicine* 15(4): 298-315.

Table 2.4: Adapted from U.S. Department of Health and Human Services, 1996, *Physical activity and health: A report of the Surgeon General* (Atlanta, GA: Centers for Disease Control and Prevention, National Center for Chronic Disease Prevention and Health Promotion) and J.F. Sallis, J.J. Prochaska and W.C. Taylor, 2000, "A review of correlates of physical activity of children and adolescents," *Medicine and Science in Sports and Exercise* 32(5): 963-975.

Table 2.8: Adapted from L.K. Bartholomew, G.S. Parcel, G. Kok and N.H. Gottlieb, 2001, *Intervention-mapping: Designing theory and evidence-based health promotion programs* (New York, NY: McGraw-Hill).

Table 3.1: Adapted from P.A. Hastie, 1998, "Skill and tactical development during sport education season," *Research Quarterly for Exercise and Sport* 69(4): 368-379.

Table 4.1: Adapted from Healthy People 2010. http://www.healthypeople.gov

Table 5.2: Adapted from Nutrition and Physical Activity Work Group, 2002, *Guidelines for comprehensive program to promote healthy eating and physical activity* (Champaign, IL: Human Kinetics).

Table 7.2: Adapted from L.K. Bartholomew, G.S. Parcel, G. Kok and N.H. Gottlieb, 2001, *Intervention mapping: Designing theory- and evidence-based health promotion programs* (New York, NY: McGraw-Hill).

Table 8.1: Adapted from R.R. Pate and J.S. Sirard, 2000, "Physical activity in young people," *Topics in Nutrition* 8(1): 1-18.

Table 8.4: Adapted from U.S. Department of Health and Human Services, 1996, *Physical activity and health: A report of the Surgeon General* (Atlanta, GA: Centers for Disease Control and Prevention, National Center for Chronic Disease Prevention and Health Promotion).

Table 9.3: Adapted from U.S. Department of Health and Human Services, 2002, *Physical activity evaluation handbook* (Atlanta, GA: Centers for Disease Control and Prevention).

Table 9.8: Adapted from U.S. Department of Health and Human Services, 2002, *Physical activity evaluation handbook* (Atlanta, GA: Centers for Disease Control and Prevention), and Health Communication Unit, 1997, *Evaluating health promotion programs* (Toronto, Canada: Centre for Health Promotion, University of Toronto).

Table 10.2: Adapted from A. Steckler and L. Linnan, Eds., 2002, *Process evaluation for public health interventions and research* (San Francisco, CA: Jossey-Bass), and T. Baranowski and G. Stables, 2000, "Process evaluation of the 5-a-day projects," *Health Education and Behavior* 27(2): 157-166.

Table 10.5: Adapted, by permission, from The Health Communication Unit at the Centre for Health Promotion, University of Toronto, 1997.

Table 10.7: Adapted from U.S. Department of Health and Human Services, 2002, *Physical activity evaluation handbook* (Atlanta, GA: Centers for Disease Control and Prevention), and Health Communication Unit, 1997, *Evaluating health promotion programs* (Toronto, Canada: Centre for Health Promotion, University of Toronto).

Figures

Figure 2.1: Adapted from A. Bandura, 1986, *Social foundations of thought and action* (New York, NY: Prentice Hall).

Figure 4.1: Adapted from the Centers for Disease Control and Prevention (CDC). Available: http://www.cdc.gov/HealthyYouth/CSHP/.

Figure 7.1: Adapted from the Centers for Disease Control and Prevention (CDC), 1999, "Framework for program evaluation in public health," *MMWR Recommendations and Reports* 48(No. RR-11): 1-40, and U.S. Department of Health and Human Services, 2002, *Physical activity evaluation handbook* (Atlanta, GA: Centers for Disease Control and Prevention). Available: http://www.cdc.gov/nccdphp/dnpa/physical/handbook.

Figure 9.1: Adapted from the Centers for Disease Control and Prevention (CDC), 1999, "Framework for program evaluation in public health," *MMWR Recommendations and Reports* 48(No. RR-11): 1-40, and U.S. Department of Health and Human Services, 2002, *Physical activity evaluation handbook* (Atlanta, GA: Centers for Disease Control and Prevention). Available: http://www.cdc.gov/nccdphp/dnpa/physical/handbook.

Figure 10.1: Adapted from the Centers for Disease Control and Prevention (CDC), 1999, "Framework for program evaluation in public health," *MMWR Recommendations and Reports* 48(No. RR-11): 1-40, and U.S. Department of Health and Human Services, 2002, *Physical activity evaluation handbook* (Atlanta, GA: Centers for Disease Control and Prevention). Available: http://www.cdc.gov/nccdphp/dnpa/physical/handbook.

NAP SACC instrument (appendix 5.A): Reprinted, by permission, from A.S. Ammerman, S.E. Benjamin, J.K. Sommers and D.S. Ward, 2004, *The Nutrition and Physical Activity Self-Assessment for Child Care (NAP SACC) environmental self-assessment instrument*, Division of Public Health, NC DHHS, Raleigh, NC, and the Center for Health Promotion and Disease Prevention, UNC-Chapel Hill, Chapel Hill, NC.

PDPAR instrument (appendix 8.A): Used with permission of Dr. Russell Pate, University of South Carolina. Adapted from A.T. Weston, R. Petosa and R.R. Pate, 1997, "Validity of an instrument for measurement of physical activity in youth," *Medicine and Science in Sports and Exercise* 29(1): 138-143.

SAPAC instrument (appendix 8.B): Reprinted, by permission, from J.F. Sallis, P.K. Strikmiller, D.W. Harsha, H.A. Feldman, S. Ehlinger, E.J. Stone, J. Williston and S. Woods, 1996, "Validation of interviewer and self-administered physical activity checklists for fifth grade students," *Medicine and Science in Sports and Exercise* 28(7): 840-851.

Appendix 8.C table: Adapted from R.W. Motl, R.K. Dishman, S.G. Trost, R.P. Saunders, M. Dowda, G. Felton, D.S. Ward and R.R. Pate, 2000, "Factorial validity and invariance of questionnaires measuring social-cognitive determinants of physical activity among adolescent girls," *Preventive Medicine* 31(5): 584-594.

Appendix 8.D table: Adapted from R.W. Motl, R.K. Dishman, R. Saunders, M. Dowda, G. Felton and R.R. Pate, 2001, "Measuring enjoyment of physical activity in adolescent girls," *American Journal of Preventive Medicine* 21(2): 110-117.

Appendix 8.E table: Adapted from J.F. Sallis, W.C. Taylor, M. Dowda, P.S. Freedson, and R.R. Pate, 2002, "Correlates of vigorous physical activity for children in grades 1 through 12: Comparing parent-reported and objectively measured physical activity," *Pediatric Exercise Science* 14(1), 30-44.

Logos

Spark: Logo courtesy of the SPARK (Sports, Play & Active Recreation for Kids) Project. © SPARK, Inc.

Take 10!: Take 10!® is a registered trademark of the ILSI Research Foundation/ Center for Health Promotion. © 2000, 2002, 2006 ILSI Research Foundation. All rights reserved.

JumpSTART: From JumpSTART, a program of the National Recreation and Park Association and the National Heart, Lung, and Blood Institute.

http://www.nhlbi.nih.gov/health/prof/heart/other/jumpstrt.htm

CATCH: CATCH and the CATCH logo are registered trademarks of the Regents of the University of California, and licensed to FlagHouse, Inc.

CHIC: Logo courtesy of the CHIC (Cardiovascular Health in Children and Youth) Study, UNC-Chapel Hill.

Pathways: Logo courtesy of the Pathways Project, University of New Mexico.

Eat Well and Keep Moving: Logo courtesy of L.W.Y. Cheung, S.L. Gortmaker and H. Dart, 2001, *Eat well and keep moving* (Champaign, IL: Human Kinetics).

TAAG: Logo courtesy of the TAAG Study. Research for this study was funded by grants from the National Heart, Lung, and Blood Institute (U01HL66858, U01HL66857, U01HL66845, U01HL66856, U01HL66855, U01HL66853, U01HL66852).

LEAP: Logo courtesy of the Lifestyle Education for Activity Project (LEAP).

NAP SACC: Logo courtesy of the NAP SACC Project, UNC-Chapel Hill.

Girls Rule!: Logo courtesy of the Girls Rule! Project, UNC Department of Nutrition.

GEMS: Logo courtesy of the GEMS Study, University of Minnesota.

PACE: Logo courtesy of the PACE (Physician-based Assessment and Counseling for Exercise) Project, © The Center for Health Interventions and Technology, LLC.

Physical Activity Behavior

one

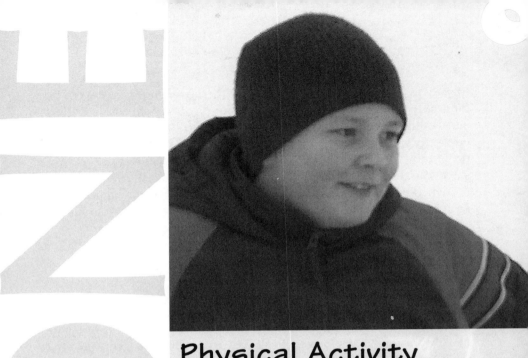

ONE

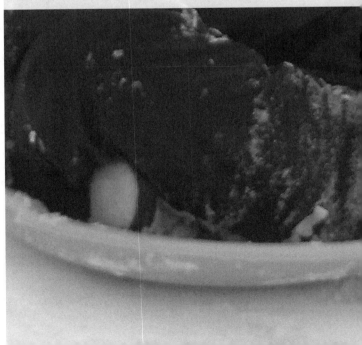

Physical Activity
Behavior Unique
to Children
and Adolescents

Physical activity might seem like a simple behavior. Indeed, we often take for granted the activity that is a part of our day-to-day lives. For children and youth, physical activity might appear to be second nature, and certainly we tend to see high levels of activity as an essential and pre-programmed component of the typical youngster's lifestyle. We might say to ourselves, "Whew! Will these little guys ever slow down?" In truth, though, physical activity is a very complex behavior. In young people, it is so complicated that researchers have only a rudimentary understanding of the factors that influence participation in physical activity.

Physical Activity Definitions

Physical activity is a complex behavior because it can be performed in many specific ways, in innumerable physical and social settings, and for many reasons. Competing in a triathlon, playing on a preschool playground, walking to a neighbor's house, mowing the lawn, and strolling from the living room to the kitchen are all forms of physical activity. Typically, physical activity is a volitional behavior that people, including children and adolescents, perform because they want or need to perform it. But sometimes we engage in physical activity because we have to: A physical education teacher might require her students to perform a series of calisthenic exercises, or a parent might require his child to walk to school. In this chapter, we define several terms often used to discuss physical activity behavior in children and youth. In addition, we discuss the major types of physical activities that are performed by young people. In so doing, we review the demographic factors that tend to be associated with physical activity in children and adolescents.

Physical Activity, Exercise, and Physical Fitness

The terms physical activity, exercise, and physical fitness are sometimes used interchangeably to describe bodily movement or programs designed to promote movement. Each of these terms, however, has a specific meaning. Physical activity is bodily movement produced by the skeletal muscles that expends energy beyond resting levels. It includes occupational activities (walking, sweeping, lifting, etc.), transportation activities (walking to work, cycling to school, etc.), recreational activities (skating, rowing, gardening, etc.), and exercise. For children, active play

4

is (or should be!) the most common form of physical activity. Exercise is physical activity that is planned, structured, repetitive, purposeful, and intended to maintain or improve health or fitness, such as step aerobics or weight training. Physical fitness is a set of attributes related to a person's ability to perform physical activity and includes cardiorespiratory fitness, strength, flexibility, and body composition.

Intensities of Physical Activity

Physical activity is performed across a remarkably wide range of intensities. It can be performed at a light, easy pace, as in strolling from store to store at a shopping mall, or it can be pursued at an exhaustive level of exertion, as with a track runner during the last lap of a race. Technically, the range of intensities available to any individual is set by his or her physical fitness level—the higher the fitness, the greater the upper limit of activity intensity. But in reality, almost all of the physical activity we perform is "submaximal" in nature. In fact, most of a young person's physical activity is performed at modest intensities.

Intensity of physical activity can be defined in technical, physiological terms or in more qualitative terms. A common nomenclature uses the terms sedentary, light, moderate, vigorous, and very vigorous to describe specific intensity zones in the continuum from rest to highly intense activity. Table 1.1 provides operational definitions of these terms and includes common examples of each physical activity intensity category. Because the health benefits of physical activity are thought to result primarily

Table 1.1 Levels of Physical Activity

ACTIVITY LEVEL	DEFINITION	EXAMPLES
Sedentary	1.0 METs*	Lying down, sitting, watching television
Light	1.1 METs-2.9 METs	Walking at 2 mph, slow cycling, stretching, light conditioning exercises
Moderate	3.0 METs-5.9 METs	Walking at 3-4.5 mph, cycling at 5-9 mph, doubles tennis
Vigorous	6.0 METs-8.9 METs	Walking at >5.0 mph, jogging, cycling at >10 mph or uphill, singles tennis
Very vigorous	>9.0 METs	Running

*MET: metabolic equivalent. 1 MET is the energy required to support the body during its resting state.

from accumulating adequate amounts of activity of at least moderate intensity, many intervention programs have been designed to increase children's and youths' participation in moderate-to-vigorous intensity physical activity, often referred to as MVPA. Physical activity guidelines for the public have often been presented in terms of daily minutes of MVPA, meaning minutes of activity at or above the threshold for moderate intensity. Recommendations for youth physical activity levels are presented later in this chapter.

Bouts of Physical Activity

It is tempting to think of children as miniature adults, but when it comes to physical activity, this is generally inappropriate. Many adults who lead physically active lives perform much of their activity in sustained periods of moderate to vigorous exercise—they jog, cycle, walk, or perform aerobics at a steady pace for 20 to 40 minutes or more. A bout of physical activity is a period of time during which the participant is active at some designated intensity level. Sustained bouts of 20 or more minutes are common in physically active adults, but they are rare in young people, particularly younger children. Figure 1.1 presents data from one study in which bouts of physical activity were monitored in children and youth of varying ages during a full week of observation (Trost et al., 2002). As shown in the figure, children more frequently engage in shorter (5-minute) bouts of physical activity than in sustained (20-minute) bouts. Young children tend to accumulate physical activity in short, sporadic bouts—they often dart from one spot to another in a few seconds, then rest briefly before darting to another spot. This form of activity is natural for young children. Adolescents, on the other hand, are more adultlike and often engage in activity that is sustained for several minutes.

This transition from play to purposeful physical activity occurs based on growth and development and is shaped by the social and physical environment within which a youngster lives. Motor skills develop as the individual grows older; infants learn to roll over, sit up, and take first steps. Children begin to throw, catch, hop, and skip. Eventually, assisted by exposure to a variety of opportunities and with appropriate encouragement, children develop the skills and interest to participate in games, sports, and recreational pursuits. Likes and preferences combine with motor skills and behavioral competencies, and the combination, if successful, results in a physically active young person.

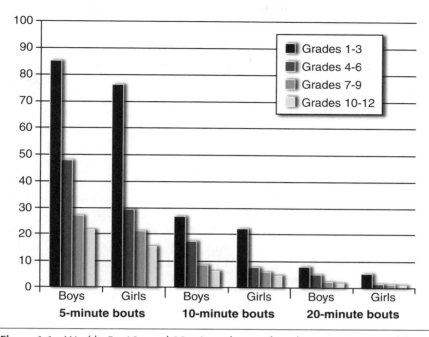

Figure 1.1 Weekly 5-, 10-, and 20-minute bouts of moderate-to-vigorous physical activity (>3 METs).

Sedentary Behavior

A sedentary activity involves little or no movement. Common examples are sleeping, watching television, reading, working at a computer, and riding in an automobile. In the past, experts tended to think of sedentary behavior as the mathematical complement of MVPA. With this mind-set, one would expect a decrease in time spent in sedentary activities to produce an increase in MVPA. However, this view tends to overlook the significance of light physical activity, the intensity zone that lies between sedentary behavior and moderate-intensity physical activity. Recent research suggests that sedentary behavior and MVPA might be much more independent of one another than previously thought. Much of a young person's day is spent in light activity, so changes in sedentary behavior or MVPA might result primarily in changes in time spent in light activity. To be more specific, reducing a child's time spent watching television might increase his or her time in light activity but is not likely to increase MVPA.

* moderate-to-vigorous intensity physical activity

Energy Expenditure

Physical activity is inextricably linked to energy expenditure. Physical activity involves work that is accomplished via contraction of the body's skeletal muscles. When muscles contract, they consume chemical energy that is made available through a lengthy set of physiological and biochemical processes. Without regard to the complexities of this system, the fundamental point is that physical activity is not possible without the expenditure of chemical energy in the muscles that are performing the activity. For example, while running across a playground, a child's leg muscles contract powerfully to drive the child's body forward. That muscular work depends on energy expended by the active muscles of the leg. Importantly, the intensity of the physical activity is directly related to the rate of energy expenditure. That is, the more intense the activity, the greater the rate of energy expenditure required to support the activity. As shown in figure 1.2, the speed of movement in walking and running is directly related to the rate at which energy is expended during the activity (Morgan et al., 2002).

Energy expenditure during physical activity is of great interest in contemporary society because of the rising prevalence of obesity. Maintenance of normal body weight requires a balance between the energy consumed from food and the energy expended throughout the day. Physical activity is a major contributor to the body's daily energy expenditure.

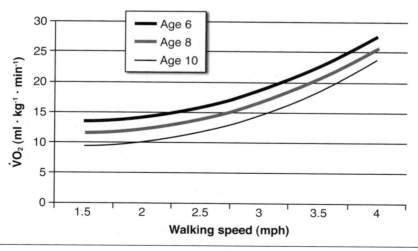

Figure 1.2 Predicted $\dot{V}O_2$ values during walking in children.

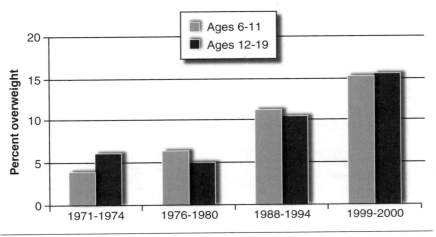

Figure 1.3 Prevalence of overweight children and youth, 1971-1974 through 1999-2000.

Consequently, people who are inactive and therefore expend relatively little energy to support physical activity are at increased risk of gaining excessive weight. Experts agree that the decreasing level of physical activity is a major factor underlying the current epidemic of obesity seen in the developed countries of the world. Figure 1.3 shows the population trend for obesity in American children and youth (National Center for Health Statistics, 2004).

Physiological Markers of Physical Activity Intensity

The increase in energy expenditure that accompanies physical activity requires an extensive array of adjustments in the body's functions. Central to these responses are marked changes in the function of the cardiovascular and respiratory systems. These two systems, working in tandem, are responsible for transporting oxygen from the atmosphere to the cells of the body. The respiratory system (including the lungs and breathing passages) moves oxygen-rich air from the atmosphere into tiny air sacs in the lungs. The cardiovascular system (including the heart and blood vessels) picks up oxygen in blood that passes through the lungs and then moves that oxygenated blood to the tissues of the body. During exercise, energy expended in the active muscles is produced with the use of oxygen, and this oxygen must be delivered to the muscles at a

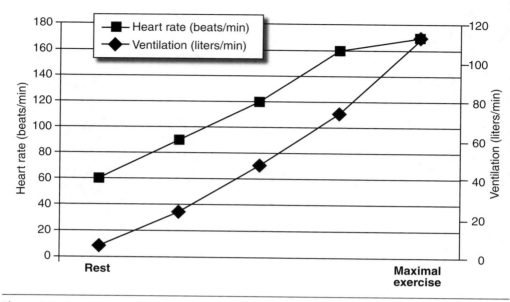

Figure 1.4 Heart rate and ventilation responses to physical activity.

rate that is directly linked to the rate of energy expenditure. If the rate of oxygen delivery falls behind the rate of energy expenditure, fatigue sets in rather quickly. Figure 1.4 shows two key responses of the cardiovascular and respiratory systems during physical activity across a wide range of intensities. As shown in the figure, the overall rate of ventilation (movement of air through the lungs) and the heart rate (frequency of the heart's contractions) are closely related to the intensity of activity. Because both ventilation and heart rate can easily be monitored by exercisers, including children and youth, these physiological factors provide important and useful guidance regarding the intensity of physical activity.

Purposes of Physical Activity

Why are children physically active? There are two basic, and perhaps obvious, answers: first, because they want to be, and second, because they have to be. Much of a child's or young person's physical activity is performed because he or she must be physically active in order to accomplish something that is seen as necessary or important. For example, if a teenage girl wants to socialize with a friend after school, she might have to walk to the friend's house. In this case, the physical activity is a means to an end, certainly not an end in itself. Also, in some cases a child is required by a supervising adult to be physically active. This would be the case in a physical education class or when children are required by parents to perform household chores such as mowing the lawn. However, a great deal of a child's physical activity is entirely volitional in nature—that is, the child is active because he or she chooses to be active. Most children, particularly those under 10 years of age, are naturally drawn to physical activity. Young children tend to move spontaneously, and physical activity is one of the major ways in which they learn about the world. For most children physical activity is fun; children can be drawn to it because the activity itself is enjoyable (it just feels good to run, bike, or swim) or because the social setting of the activity is enjoyable.

Informal Play

One definition of play is the spontaneous activity of children. Play is a very important source of physical activity and is particularly important for children and youth. The concept of play carries a connotation of freedom and choice—we play because it is fun, not because it is mandatory. Children given free time in a conducive environment tend to play spontaneously. Young children tend to play alone or in parallel with other children, while older children seek out others for organized social play activities. Not all play is physically active (e.g., board games such as checkers), but play and physical activity are usually linked. These connections among play, fun, and physical activity are central to efforts to promote physical activity in young people.

Structured Play

Much of a child's play is informal—it happens spontaneously and might include little or no adult involvement. But as children grow older, they encounter many opportunities for structured play, including youth sport programs, organized recreation and outdoor activity programs, and lessons in dance and other forms of physical activity. An estimated 30 million American children and youth participate in such programs each year, according to the National SAFE KIDS Campaign (www.safekids.org); it seems certain that these programs represent an important source of physical activity for young people in contemporary society. Many of the structured play programs available to children and youth involve competitive team sports such as soccer, basketball, and baseball. Others involve individual competitive sports such as track, swimming, gymnastics, and tennis. While such youth sport programs clearly provide many participants with substantial doses of vigorous physical activity, there are limitations or problems with some of these programs. First, not all such programs provide significant amounts of activity. For example, consider a young girl who joins a recreational soccer team. The team has one 90-minute practice and one 90-minute game per week. This girl will certainly engage in some physical activity through participating on the soccer team, but the actual activity time is unlikely to total more than 60 minutes per week. While that activity is beneficial, it does not come close to providing her with all the activity she needs on a daily basis.

Children join organized sport and physical activity programs seeking fun, social opportunities, the chance to learn new skills, and the opportunity to excel. Unfortunately, most children and youth ultimately drop out of competitive youth sport programs, often because the programs are no longer fun. According to the National Alliance for Youth Sports (www.nays.org), 70% of children drop out of organized sports by age 13. The following are the most common reasons young people drop out of programs (Stratton, 1996):

- The coach didn't understand kids.
- The coach was not a good teacher.
- I didn't get to play enough.
- There was too much emphasis on winning.
- The coach played favorites.
- I didn't like my teammates.
- The coach put too much pressure on me.

It is interesting to note that most of the reasons are related to the coach or coaching style. In other words, there are things that adults could change to increase the likelihood of children's continuing in sport programs. The message seems clear—structured physical activity programs can provide children and youth with significant amounts of MVPA, but many programs operate in ways that minimize the chances that kids will stay involved over the long term.

Transportation

We often take for granted our ability to move our bodies from place to place, that is, to transport ourselves through muscle-powered movement.

But if you consider the quality of life experienced by those who are unable to move themselves through normal muscular activity, such as patients with severe spinal cord injuries, it is clear that physical activity is a critical component of normal human existence. For children and youth, transportation is a common, important, and often enjoyable source of physical activity. Unfortunately, transportation appears to be a rapidly declining contributor to overall physical activity for children and youth in the United States and in other developed countries. Walking or riding a bike to school, once a very common and significant source of physical activity, has become a rare behavior in American children. As shown in figures 1.5 and 1.6, the percentage of American children who walk or bike to school is very low, considerably lower than for their counterparts in other countries (Centers for Disease Control and Prevention [CDC], 2001; Evenson, Hutson, McMillen, Bors, & Ward, 2003; Sirard, Ainsworth, McIver, & Pate, 2005). Even though children and younger adolescents are unable to drive an automobile, it seems clear that motorized transportation has largely replaced muscle-powered transportation as much for young people as it has for American adults.

Physical Education

Physical education, an institution in American schools for over a century, is offered in virtually all public schools in the United States. However,

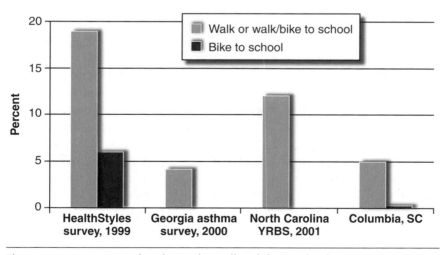

Figure 1.5 Percentage of students who walk or bike to school.

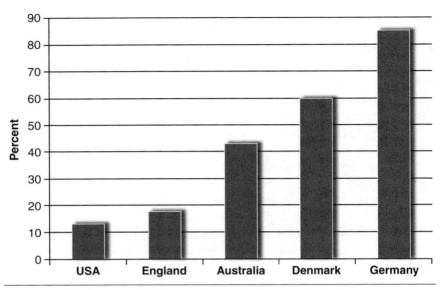

Figure 1.6 Percentage of children walking or biking to school, by country.

a student's level of exposure to physical education and the availability of professionally certified physical education teachers vary widely across states and districts. Despite this, physical education is potentially a very important provider of physical activity to the school-aged population. Its actual contribution to the physical activity levels of children and youth, though, remains a controversial issue. Some studies have shown that, on average, children receive only a few minutes of physical activity during a physical education class (National Institute of Child Health and Human Development, 2003; McKenzie et al., 1996; Stone, McKenzie, Welk, & Booth, 1998). On the other hand, large-scale studies such as Child and Adolescent Trial for Cardiovascular Health (CATCH; Luepker et al., 1996) have demonstrated that, with modified instructional practices, children can be physically active for at least half of a physical education class period. CATCH showed that the intensity of physical activity in physical education classes was significantly higher in the schools receiving the intervention program and that children in the intervention schools reported significantly more daily vigorous activity than children in the control schools (Luepker et al., 1996).

Another controversial issue is the amount of physical education that schools are required to provide students. It is clear that high school students in the United States today take fewer physical education classes than their counterparts did several decades ago. State regulations pertinent to physical education have become less rigorous and more permissive of individual district choice regarding physical education requirements. There are concerns as well that the drive to promote academic learning and to increase standardized test scores has prompted many school boards to divert resources from physical education in order to provide more funding to traditional academic areas (Sallis, McKenzie, Kolody, & Curtis, 1996; Sallis & Patrick, 1994). These trends suggest that, for various reasons, physical education is not currently realizing its potential for helping children get the physical activity they need. Data presented in table 1.2 do show an increase over the past decade in the percentage of American high school students enrolled in physical education (56% in 2003 as compared to 49% in 1991); however, only 28% of American high school students take physical education on a daily basis, significantly down from 42% in 1991 (Youth Risk Behavior Surveillance System, 2004). Other research studies indicate even lower levels of physical education enrollment in the United States, with nearly 79% of adolescents having no physical education enrollment and with only 15% of adolescents engaging in physical education five times per week (Gordon-Larsen, McMurray, & Popkin, 2000).

Work at Home and for Pay

Although we now have federal and state laws that are intended to protect children from exploitation and other risks associated with labor, it

Table 1.2   Percentage of American High School Students Enrolled in Physical Education and Taking Daily Physical Education

	ENROLLED IN PHYSICAL EDUCATION	DAILY PHYSICAL EDUCATION
2003	55.7	28.4
2001	51.7	32.2
1999	56.1	29.1
1997	48.8	27.4
1995	59.6	25.4
1993	52.1	34.3
1991	48.9	41.6

is clear that young people perform work of many types. Often the work of children and adolescents is performed at home or for a family business. Many adolescents, particularly girls, are required by their parents to supervise younger siblings after school, on weekends, and during the summers. Others assist parents with the operation of family businesses; and although family farms are less numerous than in previous decades, many youth still grow up on farms and perform farm labor from a young age. Many children also work outside the context of their families. Once they reach legal age, millions of adolescents perform work for pay (Rubenstein, Sternbach, & Pollack, 1999). Because most children and youth are not prepared to perform jobs that require advanced education or other forms of training, they tend to work in positions that involve significant doses of physical activity. Examples include yard work, child care, stocking shelves in a grocery store, and waiting tables in a restaurant. Because labor has not traditionally been considered a major source of physical activity in children and youth, we know relatively little about the impact of work-related physical activity on the total physical activity participation of young people. However, it seems very likely that, because the physical demands of work have decreased for adult laborers on average, they likely have decreased for youth as well. For example, since farming is now largely mechanized, young farm workers, though they might be quite active, are probably less active than their counterparts were in the past.

Physical Activity Guidelines

A critical question for parents, professionals, and scientists concerned with providing and promoting physical activity in young people is, How much physical activity do children and adolescents need? This might seem like a rather straightforward question for which there should be a clear and simple answer. In fact, the question is quite complicated, in part because it has several important subquestions, including, How much activity do kids need to grow and develop normally? How much is required to maintain good health and fitness during childhood and adolescence? How much activity do young people need in order to be prepared for a healthy and fit adulthood? These are important, challenging questions.

A major reason these questions are important is that the answers represent attractive and appropriate aims for physical activity interventions. Interventions to increase physical activity require goals—specific types and amounts of physical activity that are definable in terms of anticipated benefits to the young people who will be targeted in the intervention. Also, knowing how much physical activity children and adolescents need is important so that systems can be designed for monitoring physical activity levels in this population.

In recent years, physical activity guidelines for adults have been developed and extensively disseminated. The most widely accepted guideline, first presented by the U.S. Centers for Disease Control and Prevention and the American College of Sports Medicine in 1995, indicates that all adults should participate in at least 30 minutes of moderate-intensity physical activity on most days (Pate et al., 1995). This guideline was based on an expert panel's interpretation of the epidemiological studies linking habitual physical activity to risk of developing chronic diseases such as coronary heart disease. While those data are quite compelling in adults, children and adolescents rarely develop the chronic diseases that are so common later in life. Consequently, physical activity guidelines for young people cannot be based on levels of activity needed to prevent disease. Nonetheless, on the premise that youth should be at least as physically active as older persons, some agencies have applied adult guidelines to young persons. For example, the U.S. government's Healthy People 2010 (2000), a document that presents a wide range of health goals for the American population, includes the following objectives:

- Increase the proportion of adolescents who engage in moderate physical activity for at least 30 minutes on five or more of the previous seven days (Section 22-6)
- Increase the proportion of adolescents who engage in vigorous physical activity that promotes cardiorespiratory fitness three or more days per week for 20 or more minutes per occasion (Section 22-7)
- Increase the proportion of the nation's public and private schools that require daily physical education for all students (Section 22-8)
- Increase the proportion of adolescents who spend at least 50% of school physical education class time being physically active (Section 22-10)

Although epidemiological studies of physical activity and disease outcomes cannot be undertaken on young people, some scientific studies in adolescents have shown the effects of controlled exercise training on physiologic risk factors for chronic disease such as blood pressure, body fatness, and bone density. The results of these studies have been reviewed by expert panels for the purpose of establishing physical activity guidelines in young people. One such panel, the International Consensus Conference on Physical Activity Guidelines for Adolescents, was convened in San Diego in 1993. This panel issued a two-component recommendation (Sallis & Patrick, 1994):

- All adolescents should be active daily, or nearly every day, as part of play, games, sport, work, transportation, recreation, physical education, or planned exercise, in the context of family, school, and community activities.
- Adolescents should engage in three or more sessions per week of activities that last 20 minutes or more at a time and that require moderate to vigorous levels of exertion.

Another approach to establishing physical activity guidelines is based on consideration of two types of scientific evidence: current activity levels of youth and population trends for health outcomes such as obesity. It is well documented that children and adolescents in the United States and other developed countries have become fatter in recent decades (see figure 1.3). Because physical activity, along with diet, is a key determinant of body fatness, it is reasonable to conclude that the current activity level of children and youth is not sufficient to prevent the rising prevalence of obesity. This logic was applied by an international expert panel convened by the Health Education Authority of England in 1997 (Cavill, Biddle, & Sallis, 2001). After reviewing available data on population levels of physical activity, the panel concluded that most young people participate in 30 minutes of physical activity on most days, but that a great many are not active for 60 minutes daily. This observation prompted the panel to recommend a public health goal of 1 hour of at least moderate-intensity physical activity per day. The panel's specific guidelines are as follows:

- All young people should participate in physical activity of at least moderate intensity for 1 hour per day.
- Young people who currently do little activity should participate in physical activity of at least moderate intensity for at least half an hour per day.
- At least twice a week, some of these activities should help enhance and maintain muscular strength, flexibility, and bone health.

The importance of physical activity for children and adolescents is underscored in a recent review paper (Fulton, Garg, Galuska, Rattay, & Caspersen, 2004). Using Medline searches restricted to English language sources from 1980 to the present, Fulton and colleagues found that 10 organizations had developed a total of 13 public health physical activity or physical fitness recommendations. In general, the recommendations were for either 30 or 60 minutes of daily MVPA. More recent recommendations advocated 60 or more minutes of daily physical activity, probably due to the increased rates of overweight seen in today's youth (Strong et al., 2005).

SUMMARY

Physical activity is very important to the health and well-being of children and adolescents. Opportunities for activity have declined due to lowered requirements for physical education, greater reliance on motorized transportation, and attractive sedentary pursuits. Youth enjoy school and community sports but often drop out because of waning enjoyment (e.g., too much emphasis on competition and lack of fun). Rates of overweight in youth have risen, and many experts attribute much of the increase in obesity to less participation in physical activities. In order to address these deficiencies, special programs might need to be developed that focus on the unique needs of local populations. Settings such as schools, communities, or homes can be used to increase physical activity in youth as discussed in subsequent chapters.

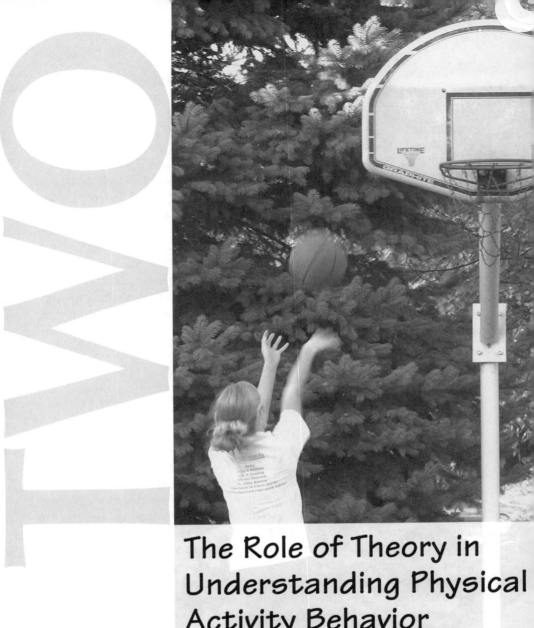

The Role of Theory in Understanding Physical Activity Behavior

Physical activity declines over childhood, and many adolescents, especially girls, engage in little physical activity. More than a decade of research has indicated that many American children and adolescents are considered to be low-active with regard to physical activity participation (Aaron et al., 1993; Baranowski, Hooks, Tsong, Cieslik, & Nader, 1987; Kann et al., 1995; Myers, Strikmiller, Webber, & Berenson, 1996; Rekers, Sanders, Strauss, Rasbury, & Morey, 1989; Dollman, Norton, & Norton, 2005). It is therefore crucial for professionals who wish to design programs for promoting physical activity in children to consider the psychosocial factors that influence activity behavior in children and youth. Successful intervention programs are devised when researchers take into account individual intention as well as environmental influences, both of which can be identified through theories and scientific studies. In this chapter, we consider theories that have been applied advantageously to improve the understanding of physical activity in children and adolescents; we also show how such theories can be employed to develop effective programs to promote physical activity in this age group.

Explaining Behavior With Theory

Why are some people not active, even though they know that physical activity is beneficial to their health? Why are some people physically active no matter what, while others cannot maintain a habit of activity? Researchers generate theories to help answer questions such as these and to provide a way to identify important influences on behavior. A theory is a set of statements or principles used primarily to explain a phenomenon but also to predict future outcomes. By identifying influences on behavior, we can design effective health promotion programs that target those influences and thereby increase physical activity. For example, if social factors such as support from family and friends are important influences on physical activity in adolescents, then providing opportunities for youths to be physically active with friends might be a more effective strategy for promoting physical activity than teaching them why they should be active.

Thinking about the behavior of people and inanimate objects dates at least as far back as Aristotle, who mused in the fourth century BC about the etiology of change in the universe. In the two dozen centuries that separate us from the ancient Greeks, however, researchers in fields such as psychology, anthropology, and philosophy have created abundant theories to explain human behavior. For example, Sigmund Freud's psy-

---

Table 2.1   Theories Used in Youth Physical Activity Studies

THEORY	HOW THEORY HAS BEEN USED
Social cognitive theory	To identify what should be included in a physical activity program (e.g., confidence and skill development) and how to design instructional school- and community-based programs
Social influences theory	To understand social influences from such groups as peers and family on physical activity and how to design programs that have social influence
Self-regulation theories	To design programs that increase participants' self-control or self-management skills necessary for being physically active
Organizational change theories	To design interventions that work with organizations such as schools or churches in a way that results in school policies and practices encouraging physical activity

Adapted from Stone, McKenzie, Welk, and Booth, 1998.

chodynamic theory held that behavior was influenced by instinct and drives operating below the level of consciousness. B.F. Skinner's radical behaviorism proposed that behavior was mainly controlled and shaped by external stimuli (Bandura, 1986).

No single theory can ever explain an entire field, especially with regard to the complex phenomenon of human behavior. For the purposes of this book, behavior theories that have been used to guide the development of youth physical activity programs or interventions, listed in table 2.1, include social cognitive theory, social influences theory, self-regulation theories, and organizational change theories. The most widely used theory for understanding physical activity, however, is social cognitive theory, which has been formally developed by researchers over the course of several decades. We therefore discuss this theory in depth. Although measurement and evaluation tools are also guided by behavior theories, explanations of how to design these tools are provided in chapter 8, "Measuring Physical Activity."

Defining Social Cognitive Theory

According to a report by the Surgeon General in 1996, social cognitive theory, largely the result of Albert Bandura's work (1986), is one of the most successful theories commonly used to guide the development of physical activity programs in youth. Bandura became disenchanted with behaviorist and determinist theories positing that the environment causes an individual's behavior. Rather than seeing a unidirectional influence, Bandura believed that the environment and the individual affected one another in a process he called *reciprocal determinism.* One model of the idea of reciprocal determinism is triadic reciprocality (figure 2.1), in which three broad factors influence one another: cognitive or personal factors within the individual, behavioral skills of the individual, and environmental factors. Bandura's idea of triadic reciprocality is quite useful for understanding the nature of physical activity. That is, to understand or influence an individual's physical activity behavior, one must consider that person's experiences, current behavioral skills, and the context or setting in which the person is expected to be active.

A theory such as social cognitive theory helps us understand behavior by partitioning it into a set of associated concepts called constructs and by illustrating how the constructs relate to each other and to behavior (Glanz, Rimer, & Lewis, 2002). Constructs are usually developed or adopted for a specific theory and take on meaning only within the context of a given theory applied to a specific situation. Consider the example in table 2.2. The first column lists a construct called perceived self-efficacy, a central concept in social cognitive theory (Bandura, 1986). This construct and its implications become much more meaningful when applied to a specific behavior such as physical activity in a specific situation.

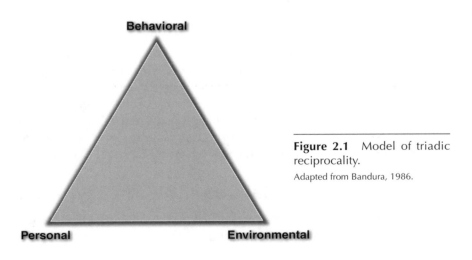

Figure 2.1 Model of triadic reciprocality.

Adapted from Bandura, 1986.

Table 2.2 How Theory Is Used to Explain Behavior

CONSTRUCT	BEHAVIOR	SITUATION
Perceived self-efficacy defined	Perceived self-efficacy applied to physical activity	How self-efficacy promotes physical activity behavior
A person's belief in his or her ability to perform a particular behavior, including confidence to overcome barriers to engaging in that behavior.	A high school girl's belief about her ability to be physically active after school even if her friends want to hang out at the mall instead.	If the high school girl is a person with high perceived self-efficacy for physical activity, she is more likely to be active even when barriers arise, such as when her friends want her to hang out at the mall with them.

Numerous constructs for understanding and changing behavior have been formulated for social cognitive theory by Bandura and others (Bandura, 1986; Mischel, 1973). Of particular interest for people who want to design physical activity programs are those constructs associated with the reciprocality model as already defined (figure 2.1). Constructs from each of the three factors (cognitive, behavioral, and environmental) in the reciprocality model are first presented in table 2.3 and then defined.

Cognitive Factors

One of the most important cognitive constructs within the individual is perceived self-efficacy, or the individual's belief that he or she can successfully engage in a given behavior (Bandura, 1986), which can also be thought of as confidence. Personal experiences, particularly perceptions of success or failure, are the largest influence on perceived self-efficacy (Bandura, 1986). A person who is confident of success is more likely to undertake a task and more likely to persist when the inevitable frustrations arise. As noted in the example given in table 2.2, a student who is confident that she can be active after school will be more likely to initiate being active after school and to solve problems when barriers present themselves. A person with low confidence might not even try, will get discouraged easily if things do not go perfectly, and will most likely quit trying when barriers arise.

Table 2.3 Constructs in Social Cognitive Theory

BROAD FACTORS OR CONSTRUCTS	SPECIFIC CONSTRUCTS	WHAT THE CONSTRUCT MEANS
Cognitive or personal factors	Perceived self-efficacy	A person's belief about his or her ability to be successful in initiating and continuing a specific activity.
	Expected outcome	A person's belief about what will happen if he or she engages in a specific activity (i.e., positive and negative consequences of being physically active).
	Coping	How a person deals with emotional (e.g., fear of failure or embarrassment) or physiological arousal (e.g., misinterpreting the normal physiological response to physical activity).
Behavioral factors	Self-control (sometimes called behavioral skills)	The ability of the individual to manage his or her own behavior including setting goals, monitoring and adjusting a plan based on what works, and using self-reinforcement (e.g., rewarding oneself when goals are reached).
	Motor or sport skills (called behavioral capability)	Having skills needed to engage in the behavior itself (e.g., being able to dance or having specific sport skills).
Environmental factors	Social environment in which the behavior takes place (e.g., social norms, social support, role model)	Family members, other adults, best friends, and peers have some influence on physical activity behavior (e.g., encouraging or discouraging it and providing such assistance as transportation).
	Physical environment in which the behavior takes place	Opportunity and safe access to a facility or program are needed to enable a motivated person to be physically active (e.g., sidewalks to school, sport programs with open enrollment).

Other individual factors related to physical activity include outcome expectations, perceived benefits (useful in adolescents, but not younger children), and perceived barriers (Sallis, Prochaska, & Taylor, 2000). Outcome expectations are what we think will happen if we are physically active. An example of a negative expectation is, "Being active after school will interfere with my social life." A positive expectation is, "Being active will help make me better in sports." Perceived benefits and barriers are specific types of beliefs about being physically active. Adolescents who expect benefits from being physically active are more likely to be active. Similarly, children and adolescents who perceive barriers to being physically active are less likely to be active.

Behavioral Factors

Self-control, the ability to manage one's own behavior or behavioral skills, has also been shown to be a very important influence on behavior (Kahn et al., 2002). The behavioral skills referred to here include goal setting, self-monitoring, problem solving, self-adjusting, and self-reward. Collectively, self-control refers to how well an individual monitors and manages his or her own behavior. For example, a high school student might set a goal to walk after school three times per week. The student would then monitor her behavior using a diary or checklist to keep track of her after-school walking. If her goal was not being met, she would make adjustments in her plan, based on the barriers encountered. She also would acknowledge her success when she has reached her goal (self-reward or self-reinforcement). This approach is more effective with adolescents and older youth who have the cognitive ability to develop plans and anticipate consequences than it is with younger children.

Environmental Factors

In social cognitive theory, environment refers to any factor outside the individual and includes both the physical and the social environment. For children, spending time outdoors is often associated with being physically active (Sallis et al., 2000). The social environment, especially the influence of family and peers, has also been shown to be an important influence on physical activity in children and adolescents (U.S. Department of Health and Human Services [DHHS], 1996; Sallis et al., 2000). Children are more active if parents provide encouragement and transportation and if their parents are active with them (Gustafson & Rhodes, 2006). Adolescents are more active if they have assistance and support for being active from their parents, as well as support from significant others (Sallis et al., 2000). The environment is an important influence on physical activity in children and adolescents, particularly in regard to access to physical activity opportunities.

Applying Behavior Theory

Theory can help us understand physical activity behavior. However, the usefulness of a theory is demonstrated when the theory is applied in "real world" settings to change physical activity behavior. Fortunately, many theories and their respective constructs used in physical activity research have been tested in programs, and experts have identified those that are the most important. So what does influence children to be active, and what influences them to be physically inactive? Summaries of the key influences on physical activity in youth and related theory constructs are presented in table 2.4.

Identifying the "Right" Theory

This book uses a problem-driven approach rather than a theory-driven approach (Bartholomew, Parcel, Kok, & Gottlieb, 2001). That is, we are interested in applying what is already known from theory and scientific studies to successfully promote physical activity in a particular population and setting. For example, we want to select theory based on what is most likely to get young people physically active after school time—we want to know what "works." In the problem-driven approach, the emphasis is on results, so it is common to choose some constructs from several theories. In a sense, all theories are "right" in some situation; the challenge is to find the best combination of theory constructs to apply to the specific situation. In contrast, the theory-driven approach is focused on developing or testing theory (Bartholomew et al., 2001). Researchers using the theory-driven approach are more interested in the theory itself than in increasing physical activity per se, and would likely use all of the constructs that belong in the theory being tested.

Organizing Influences Into an Ecological Model

As shown in table 2.4, many important influences on physical activity in children and adolescents have already been identified by experts. This is a rather large number of influences from which to select! Fortunately, if these influences are categorized into different levels, they can be

Table 2.4 A Summary of the Major Influences on Physical Activity in Youth

WHAT MAKES KIDS ACTIVE?	WHAT MAKES KIDS INACTIVE?	RELATED THEORY CONSTRUCTS
Having fun, enjoyment	Not enjoying it, finding it boring	*
Intending to be active		Behavioral intention
Getting something out of it; benefits (such as weight control)	Perceiving more "negatives" than benefits (e.g., not liking to get sweaty)	Beliefs, outcome expectations
Feeling able or competent	Not feeling able or competent	Perceived self-efficacy
Exploring new things, interest		*
Having the skills to be successful		Behavioral skills, behavioral capability
It's the thing to do		Social norm
Being able to do it with friends	Having no one to be active with	Social support
Receiving encouragement from family or friends		Social support
Receiving tangible assistance from adults (parents enroll children, pay for programs, provide transportation)		Social support
Emulating teacher, coach, or older students		Role model
Provision by school (or other organizations) of attractive opportunities for physical activity		Organizational policies or practices
Attractive physical activity programs or equipment available and accessible	Programs not available or not accessible	Community/ Environment— opportunity and access
Spending time outdoors (for children)	Attractive sedentary pursuits	*

*Sometimes useful constructs have been identified without a larger theoretical structure.

Adapted from U.S. Department of Health and Human Services, 1996, and Sallis, Prochaska, and Taylor, 2000.

organized in such a way that it becomes easier to select among them. For example, such influences as confidence operate from inside the individual; others such as social support originate with friends and family; and opportunities for physical activity in the community are factors outside the individual. Many experts organize these influences into levels using an ecological model, which helps to categorize the constructs from multiple theories into individual (also called intrapersonal), interpersonal, organizational, environmental or community, and policy levels of influence, as shown in figure 2.2 (McLeroy, Bibeau, Steckler, & Glanz, 1988).

An ecological model emphasizes the importance of considering multiple levels of influence and the role of the environment on behavior (Sallis & Owen, 2002). Some environments, whether social or physical, are not conducive to physical activity, while some environments have been designed to encourage activity. In addition, the ecological model can provide an effective way to organize theory constructs for a prob-

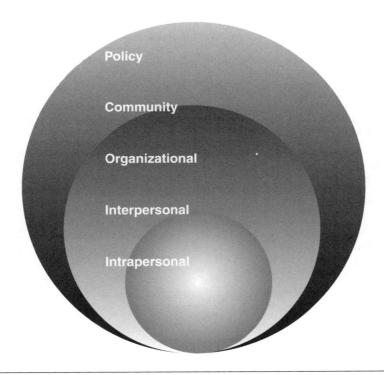

Figure 2.2 The ecological model of influence.

lem-driven approach to changing behavior (Bartholomew et al., 2001). Experts recommend using a multilevel approach to understand and promote physical activity, which means that influences on physical activity other than individual influences should be considered. Table 2.5 presents important theory constructs organized by level of influence.

Table 2.5 Ecological Approach to Organizing Constructs From Theories

LEVEL	CONSTRUCTS FROM THEORIES (INFLUENCES ON BEHAVIOR)	INCREASED ACTIVITY COMES WHEN:
Individual: influences that directly affect the individual	• Perceived self-efficacy • Expectations (including perceived benefits and barriers) • Intention to be physically active • Behavioral skills • Behavioral capability	Individuals • have confidence in their ability to be active • expect benefits from being active • intend to be active • have the behavioral skills needed to get and stay active
Interpersonal: influences from relationships, or the way people interact in small groups, or both	• Social environment (including modeling and observational learning) • Social support/Social network • Social influence approaches	Significant others • Family provides instrumental support (such as transportation). • Friends are active together. • Adults support, encourage, and model physical activity.
Organizational: influences from organizations in which children spend time (e.g., schools)	• Organizational change • Policies	The school and other organizations • provide access to fun opportunities and • have policies that support physical activity Staff are skilled at engaging youth in fun physical activity.

(continued)

Table 2.5 *(continued)*

LEVEL	CONSTRUCTS FROM THEORIES (INFLUENCES ON BEHAVIOR)	INCREASED ACTIVITY COMES WHEN:
Community/Environmental: influences from the community and environment in which children or adolescents live or spend their time	• Interorganizational relations • Community development • Advocacy approaches	The community • provides safe access to fun physical activity opportunities • reduces barriers to existing facilities and opportunities • creates new facilities and additional opportunities

Because there are multiple levels of influence on physical activity in youth, multilevel interventions or programs that target these influences are more likely to be effective in changing behavior than those that do not, assuming that resources are sufficient to implement a multilevel program (Sallis, Pinski, Grossman, Patterson, & Nader, 1988; Sallis et al., 2000). In other words, a program based on a single level of influence, such as teaching motor or sport skills for being physically active, is less likely to succeed in changing physical activity behavior than a program that carefully targets multiple levels of influence, such as teaching sport skills, increasing support from friends and family, and providing access (e.g., transportation or defrayed enrollment costs) to fun activity programs.

Using Theory
to Facilitate Behavior Change

Using theory to change behavior is most effective within the context of program planning and is one of the steps required for program planning—but not the first step. As a part of program planning, selection of a theory should be based on the population to be served, the site of program activities, the type of physical activity, and the objectives of the program. For example, a program might seek to involve young children or adolescents in sport or dance in physical education class during the school day or in a community center after school. Chapter 7 addresses the details of program planning; here we present the steps of program planning that apply to selecting theories. In order to help guide program planning, one should take the following four steps: (1) identify the specific physical activity behavior, the population, and the setting; (2) list the most important influences on the physical activity behavior; (3) select theoretical methods to be used; and (4) develop strategies that will be used in the program. These steps are discussed in detail next.

Theory Selection in Four Steps

Step 1: Identify behavior

Step 2: List influences

Step 3: Select methods

Step 4: Develop strategies

Step 1: Identify Behavior

A successful program will identify not only the specific physical activity behavior to be changed, but also the youth to be targeted (e.g., high school girls or fourth graders) in a specific setting (e.g., school or community). As already noted, details of selecting theories, methods, and strategies will vary depending on the physical activity behavior, the target group, and the setting.

Step 2: List Influences

It is important to understand the influences on the physical activity behavior of your target group. This information can be gleaned from at least two sources: review of published studies and research on behavior theory (Bartholomew et al., 2001). Practitioners and researchers often rely on professional experience as well. For example, the influences within the multilevel ecological context as described in table 2.5 are helpful for choosing the appropriate theory constructs to use in planning a program, but it is important to supplement these constructs with a current literature review, specifically with regard to your target population and setting. As already noted, table 2.4 lists the most important influences on physical activity behavior in children and adolescents based on current literature (DHHS, 1996; Sallis et al., 2000).

It is probably unrealistic to try to include in a program all the influences on physical activity that can be identified. Ideally, some aspect of behavioral influence should be selected from each of the four ecological levels shown in table 2.5. However, available resources must be taken into account. It is important to take care in considering the potential impact of community and environmental influences. Although community and environmental factors are often thought to be beyond the scope of programs or resources, these two sets of influences might be among the most critical factors in supporting behavior changes in youth. The process for setting priorities among and within ecological levels is discussed further in chapter 7.

Step 3: Select Methods

The term method, as used here, is a general term for what will be done in the physical activity program to influence physical activity behavior. This method of behavior change is the link between an influence on behavior and an intervention action designed to change that influence (Bartholomew et al., 2001). In contrast to the specific strategies used in programs (step 4), methods usually consist of general approaches that are linked with theories. Tables 2.6 and 2.7 provide a list of methods that are typically associated with theoretical constructs (Bartholomew et al., 2001). For example, if you have selected the construct of perceived self-efficacy based on the needs of your program, you would consider the general methods outlined in table 2.6 and would review the considerations for use. The use of theoretical constructs to identify important influences on behavior guides the selection of general methods based on those theoretical constructs. However, these methods do not include specific details about what to do in a program. Selecting practical strategies is the next step.

Step 4: Develop Strategies

Practical strategies that will be used in the program must be developed. This activity is the creative step between theory and practice and is the step at which planning becomes reality. A strategy is a specific action, such as using a videotape to demonstrate a specific skill. Using a videotape, for example, can aid in skill development and is an example of modeling. Not to be confused with the creation of models such as the ecological model discussed earlier, the term modeling is used in social cognitive theory to refer to a psychological process of learning as noted in table 2.6. Humans are unique in that we are capable of abstraction

Table 2.6 General Methods Associated With Theoretical Constructs at the Individual Level of Influence

Theoretical constructs	• Perceived self-efficacy • Behavioral skills • Behavioral capability
General methods suggested by theory	• Modeling—a model demonstrates the task or skill • Guided practice with feedback—students practice the task or skill with direction and feedback from the leader • Goal setting—students set realistic goals • Reinforcement—students learn how to reward themselves for reaching goals
Program objective	To increase self-efficacy, behavioral capability, and behavioral skills
Considerations for use	• Guided practice must include demonstration of the components of a skill and participant practice with feedback. • Feedback and reinforcement must be provided to the individual, should be provided immediately, and should be very specific. • Participant practice should be repeated until mastery of the skill is achieved. • Goal setting requires commitment to a goal—a goal that is difficult yet realistic given the individual's level of skill. • Modeling requires attention to and perception of relevant aspects of modeled behavior; ability to remember modeled information; and skills to translate modeled information into action. • Model should be similar to participants, should represent good effort rather than perfection, and should be reinforced or rewarded for desired outcome.
Theoretical constructs	• Expectations—for example, perceived benefits and barriers • Intention to be physically active
General methods suggested by theory	• Verbal persuasion—talking participants into it • Modeling with vicarious reinforcement—participants see model getting rewarded or reinforced
Program objective	To increase intentions and positive expectations and to reduce negative expectations
Considerations for use	Verbal persuasion must be credible, because people prefer outcomes that are likely and desirable over those that are unlikely and undesirable. Information about the desired behavior should match the young person's life and be personally relevant.

Table 2.7 General Methods Associated With Theoretical Constructs at the Interpersonal, Organizational, and Community/Environmental Levels of Influence

Interpersonal	
Theoretical constructs	• Social environment • Social norms • Social support/Social network
General methods suggested by theory	• Modeling—participants see others who are physically active and are rewarded for it • Making physical activity the "cool" thing to do • Using and strengthening existing social networks (getting family and friends to support physical activity) • Developing social support from new sources (getting support from new friends and adults)
Program objectives	• To create social environments that support physical activity • To develop or enhance social support for physical activity
Considerations for use	• See modeling details in table 2.6. • Social support requires enlisting existing network or mobilization of new network. • Consider types of support needed: emotional, instrumental, informational, appraisal. • Determine how support will be mobilized; for example, teach students how to develop support networks, or work with parents directly to create support. • Skill training for developing social support may be needed.
Organizational	
Theoretical constructs	• Organizational change • Policy change
General methods suggested by theory	Working with organizations to make changes in how they do business
Program objective	To create organizations with policies and practices that support physical activity
Considerations for use	• Requires attention to stages of organizational change • Must have skills needed to facilitate change • Must allow time for long and complex change process

Community/Environment	
Theoretical constructs	• Interorganizational relations • Advocacy approaches
General methods suggested by theory	• Working with groups of organizations to increase collaboration and change how the organizations do business with each other • Using media approaches to advocate for changes in policy • Using a variety of strategies to advocate for changes in policy
Program objective	To create communities and environments that provide opportunities and safe access to physical activity
Considerations for use	• Partnership and coalition development require attention to stages of coalition development. • Coalition members must have skills needed to facilitate change. • Coalitions need time for long and complex change process. • Advocacy approaches must match the advocacy group's style and tactics with the issue and community. • Access to media is needed for advocacy work.

and learning by observation. A significant amount of social learning is influenced by people who are around us, both in person and through such media as television. Modeling is thus a key element in many programs that seek to influence physical activity behavior; one modeling strategy just referred to is the use of a videotape. Other modeling strategies include using live demonstrations by teachers or coaches, demonstrations by students themselves, and scripted or unscripted role playing with students.

Your choice of the most appropriate strategy depends on a number of factors. In the case of skill development, although you aim to teach one specific skill, you might use others depending on who the target audience is and the setting in which the program occurs. For example, modeling strategies might be used to teach CPR skills, but these would differ from strategies used to teach students the skills of self-reinforcement or self-reward to maintain physical activity behavior. Age and skill level of the intended audience will influence how effective your approach will be, as will such constraints of the setting as lack of class time.

A good way to develop effective strategies is through review of published literature—reading about what others have done successfully.

Unfortunately, details about strategy selection are often not included in published reports. We have therefore provided in table 2.8 (adapted from Bartholomew et al., 2001) some examples of strategies that others have used. Note, though, that sometimes the best source for useful strategies is the individual creativity of the program planner.

Avoiding Common Mistakes When Using Theory

It is important to consider theory and models when developing physical activity programs for children and adolescents. However, because physical activity is a complex phenomenon, it can be difficult at times to select and apply a theoretical orientation. Some common mistakes people make when using theory to change physical activity behavior include identifying too narrow or too broad a focus for their program; selecting too few constructs or selecting constructs that do not apply well to their target group; and relying solely on their intuition to devise a program rather than reviewing published studies and other literature. The following are common problems in the design of physical activity programs:

1. Focusing program too narrowly for expected outcomes. If the purpose of the program is to change or maintain physical activity behavior, methods and strategies that focus only on providing information or increasing awareness of physical activity are probably inadequate. Such methods and strategies will likely not increase a child's or adolescent's participation in daily physical activity.

2. Selecting too few constructs. As already noted, selecting constructs at only one level of influence or not selecting enough constructs might jeopardize the success of a program. Within the resources available, a program should be based on the important influences on the behavior. It is important to remember that a program can be well executed but still miss the mark if the planning phase did not identify the important influences on the behavior.

3. Focusing too broadly in relation to the resources available. If you attempt to do too much with limited resources, your program is less likely to succeed. This problem is the opposite of the first problem listed. It involves a failure to realistically assess what is needed to carry

Table 2.8 Examples of Creative and Practical Strategies

INTENDED PURPOSE	GENERAL METHODS	EXAMPLES OF CREATIVE STRATEGIES
Individual		
Increase intention to be active Increase positive expectations of activity Reduce negative expectations	Modeling activity with positive reinforcement provided	• Show videotapes of role models (other youth) with reinforcement for being active. • Have role models describe positive experiences (testimonials). • Role models talk about their positive activity experiences (e.g., teen athletes).
Increase perceived self-efficacy Increase behavioral skills	Modeling Skill training using guided practice with feedback	• Teachers or leaders demonstrate and teach skills (such as overcoming barriers and time management) in small groups. • Participants evaluate videotaped vignettes. • Participants practice skill in pairs with feedback.
Interpersonal		
Increase social support	Increasing social support from existing sources	• Teach individual students to ask for help in being active. • Form activity buddies within student groups. • Involve parents directly in mother-daughter or father-son physical activity events.
Organizational		
Change organizations into positive influences Increase opportunities for physical activity	Planned organizational change	• Form school committee that is authorized to assess and make recommended changes to school policies and practices that affect opportunities for activity for all students.
Community		
Change community or physical environment Increase physical activity opportunities and access	Partnership development	• Work with several organizations (e.g., city recreation, local Y, or school district) on the common goal of providing fun and accessible after-school physical activity programs for youth.

Adapted from Bartholomew, Parcel, Kok, and Gottlieb, 2001.

out the program or a failure to set priorities that reflect the size of the budget.

4. Failure to consider the particular situation and target group. Using theory or constructs just because they have been used in the past fails to consider your specific population. The target group of interest, the setting for the program, and the physical activity behavior focus must be the starting points for planning. What worked well for one group in one setting might not be applicable to a similar group in another setting.

5. Using constructs from theories without considering implications. Selection of theoretical constructs should be systematic and should be based on important influences on physical activity. Ideally, the constructs should be selected from multiple levels of influence, as with the ecological model.

6. Overreliance on familiar methods or strategies. Theories that explain individual rather than interpersonal or environmental influences have been around the longest and are often the theories with which people are most comfortable. However, these are not necessarily the most applicable to behavior change.

7. Overreliance on a favorite theory. Because there are multiple influences on the suite of behaviors that influence physical activity, a single theory is unlikely to be effective for all applications.

8. Dismissing theory and relying on experience or intuition. Although some theories might seem to be intuitive, using an unexamined theory as the guiding framework for a program might not work because it is undefined and untested.

SUMMARY

Understanding the psychological, social, and environmental factors that influence the behavior of children and adolescents is a crucial aspect in designing any physical activity intervention. The main purpose of theories in social science is to explain; for physical activity, this means that we are interested in the ways in which internal and external factors affect children's and adolescents' behavior in regard to physical activity. Social cognitive theory has been invaluable to those designing health-related interventions because it combines personal, behavioral, and environmental factors in explaining change and motivation, and because the constructs that have been developed for this theory are extremely useful for designing physical activity research studies and interventions. In order to understand and apply theory in your own work, it is important to identify the behavior you wish to change, list any social or environmental influences on that behavior, select your methods carefully, and develop successful strategies through a review of published literature. Once you understand theories, constructs, ecological models, methods, and strategies, you can use Worksheet 2.1 in the appendix to select and employ behavior theories to begin planning your physical activity program for children and adolescents.

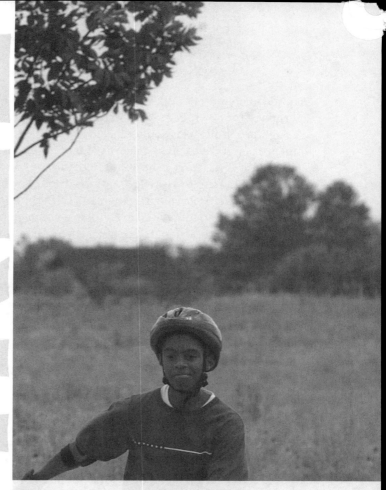

THREE

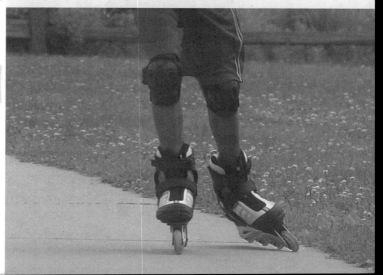

Physical Activity
Behavior Intervention

As noted in chapters 1 and 2, physical activity behavior in young people is determined by a complex set of factors, including personal characteristics (e.g., age, sex, body weight), social environments (e.g., parents, teachers, siblings, friends), and physical environments (e.g., home, neighborhood, school). Areas such as school, a child's home, or a neighborhood are called settings, or the physical location where children might participate in physical activity. Because elements of both the social and the physical environment are so influential in shaping a young person's physical activity behavior, it is important to consider the settings in which young people spend most of their time and the ways in which intervention activities in these areas can be organized for optimal results. In this chapter, we first present in detail the three major settings for intervention programs and then provide tools and suggestions that you can use to identify and organize activities in designing an intervention that will be successful in your chosen setting.

Types of Settings

Home, school, and the community are settings for youth interventions. School includes both the regular school day environment and the setting of organized after-school programs. Community is a big umbrella, but here it is broadly defined to include community agencies, religious organizations, parks, and private businesses such as fitness centers, dance studios, and martial arts gyms. Home is the setting of programs designed to be conducted at home or those initiated by the family when a child has a special condition, such as obesity. Although clinical settings are typically community based, youth generally see medical providers in association with a family member, and any intervention or "prescription" is implemented in association with someone from the home.

Home

The home environment is thought to be most important in shaping a child's physical activity behavior; however, evidence of the specific influence of family members or the physical environment is limited due to inadequate research conducted in this area (Gustafson & Rhodes, 2006). Not only do youth, particularly young children, spend much of their time in the home, but it is in the home that they associate with their parents and siblings—perhaps the most important social influences on children's activity patterns. However, today's children may not be as physically active at home as previous generations. Clearly, the typical American home today is very different from homes of the last century or even the last decade, with varied family structures such as two working parents, single-parent households, and blended families (Federal Interagency Forum on Child and Family Statistics [FIFCFS], 2005). In fact, children spend less time at home than in years past (Sturm, 2005).

Far fewer homes today are located on farms or in rural areas; most homes are now situated in urban or suburban neighborhoods that often present major barriers to physical activity. Unsafe neighborhoods with few parks and no sidewalks tend to discourage physical activity (Centers for Disease Control and Prevention, 2005). Unfortunately, those charac- teristics are highly prevalent in a great many American neighborhoods (Gordon-Larsen, Nelson, Page, & Popkin, 2006). The environment inside the home has also changed in ways that tend to make sedentary behav- ior very attractive to children and adolescents. American homes have become electronic entertainment centers: Televisions with numerous channels, video games, computers, and the Internet are literally every- where in many homes (Roberts, Foehr, & Rideout, 2005). On average, children spend more than 6 hours exposed to some type of media every day (Roberts et al., 2005). When parents fail to regulate their children's access to these forms of entertainment, there may be little inducement for the children to go outside, to find friends, and to play actively.

Another change, one that is not for the better in terms of physical activity, involves the social environment in our homes. In most American homes, both parents (or the only parent in one-parent families) work outside the home (FIFCFS, 2005). Many children thus become "latch key kids" after school, staying inside until a parent returns from work rather than going outside and playing actively. Estimates are that between 2 and 7 million American youth are "latch key kids" (Wetzstein, 2000). This living pattern can severely restrict a child's opportunity to be active during a critical time of day. Moreover, there may be special needs (e.g., among children who are obese) for which families need to seek outside guidance so that homes can be more supportive of physical activity.

School

Young people spend a high proportion of their days in school—second only to the amount of time they are at home. On average, children spend about 6.6 hours per day, or 1140 hours per year, in school; this figure increased 20 minutes per day between 1987 and 1999 (U.S. Department of

Education, 2005). The school day is, for the most part, a sedentary period in a young person's daily routine. In the traditional classroom, a high priority is given to order and quiet. Students are expected to remain seated and focused on learning. Exceptions are physical education classes, recess or other break times, and transitions between classrooms. Each of these opportunities for physical activity has been reduced, limited, and threatened in recent years (U.S. Department of Health and Human Services [DHHS], 2004; Lowry, Wechsler, Kann, & Collins, 2001; Sindelar, 2002). Physical education requirements in many schools have been reduced, and concerns have been raised that a very limited amount of physical activity is provided in many physical education classes (DHHS, 2004). Recess in elementary schools may be experiencing the same fate as physical education in high schools (Sindelar, 2002). Some schools have reduced or eliminated recess in an effort to increase classroom instruction time. Despite these disquieting trends, it is possible for students to be quite physically active during the school day, and schools play an important role in providing interscholastic sport opportunities for students at the high school level.

Communities

Many community-based settings offer opportunities for young people to be physically active. These include public recreation centers, parks, youth service organizations (e.g., YMCAs, YWCAs, Boys & Girls Clubs), commercial businesses (e.g., dance studios, karate clubs), and religious organizations. These settings provide opportunities for both unstructured and structured physical activity. Community settings are critical to young people's physical activity behavior because these settings are typically accessible at times when physical activity is available and encouraged—after school, on weekends, and during summer breaks. In addition, youth with special health needs may receive physical activity through medical facilities such as doctors' offices, hospitals, or other health care settings.

Though most communities have numerous settings in which youth can be physically active, not all children make extensive use of them. Factors that can limit a child's use of existing community-based opportunities include transportation, program cost, program offerings, and safety. If a setting is easy for children to reach and is safe and affordable for them, there is a good chance that they will be active in that setting, especially if the activities are fun and if their friends are taking part. For example, studies have shown that having parks and green spaces nearby is related to higher rates of physical activity for many children and adolescents (Sallis & Glanz, 2006). Lack of transportation to programs or play areas limits participation, especially among minority children (Gordon-Larsen et al., 2004; Hoefer, McKenzie, Sallis, Marshall, & Conway, 2001). And, if a setting is perceived as unsafe, if the available programs are not enjoyable, if the cost is prohibitive, or if transportation is unavailable, the child probably will not be active in that setting.

After-school care facilities have become a very important community setting for physical activity for children between the ages of 5 and 12. Such children are too young to be unsupervised after school, so millions of them spend the hours from 3 p.m. to 6 p.m. in after-school programs operated by public, private nonprofit, or private for-profit organizations. Between 1981 and 1997, children's discretionary time declined about 12%, or 7 to 8 hours per week (Sturm, 2005). This loss of free time is directly related to increases in time spent in school or child care (Sturm, 2005). These after-school programs vary widely in their provision of physical activity to the children they serve. Some programs provide plenty of time for free play in settings that encourage physical activity and offer special programs such as gymnastics and dance instruction. Other programs offer limited access to active play environments and allow kids to watch TV or videos for much of their time in the facility. Children in the latter type of program are unlikely to participate in much after-school physical activity.

Interaction of Home, School, and Community Settings

Today's homes provide unlimited access to multiple forms of media, including TV, video games, and computers, increasing children's potential for sedentary pursuits. However, the home setting could be a rich opportunity for family-based physical activity engagement. But, as already discussed, children spend less time at home than in past years. Less time at home means more time spent elsewhere, such as school and community. As time in structured settings at school or in the community increases, so does the importance of these settings for providing physical activity (Sturm, 2005). Physical activity levels of many youth are inadequate and could benefit from increased opportunities regardless of the setting. Intervention programs that take place in each of these settings are covered in subsequent chapters of this book.

Choosing an Intervention Setting

Public health interventions target groups rather than individuals. Thus, most physical activity interventions for youth are designed as organized programs that take place in school or community settings. Interventions that target children in school might involve training teachers to incorporate more physical activity into the school day or encouraging better use of physical education class time so that children participate in more physical activity. Interventions that target communities might involve working with a neighborhood to design safer walking and biking trails or creating a new preschool program for area children. Through such programs, children or adolescents participate in activities that result in greater amounts of health-producing physical activity.

Well-planned physical education interventions can be used as guides for designing other group activity programs, and tips for planning effective programs can be taken from these successful interventions. School is the most common setting for youth interventions, and in chapter 4 we discuss several published interventions that targeted children in a school setting. Community settings have also been used in intervention design, and in chapter 5 we provide some examples from published studies. Finally, examples of projects that have targeted youth in a home or health care setting are presented in chapter 6.

Regardless of the setting that an intervention focuses on, it is important to develop a plan for your desired outcome, or for how your program will increase physical activity among youth. Physical activity interventions can focus on two broad outcomes: increasing physical activity during the program time or increasing physical activity behavior outside of the program. In the sections that follow, we present examples of ways to increase physical activity both inside and outside of the program.

Organizing Activities

One way interventions help youth obtain more physical activity is through engagement in an active program. Organized programs may be part of the physical education curriculum, a before-school class, an after-school program at the YMCA, or a special program sponsored through a local church or synagogue. However, for many children, physical activity classes amount to waiting, sitting, or making transitions between activities, resulting in relatively little time being active. Some estimates suggest that students in physical education classes spend as few as 10 minutes engaged in moderate activities like walking and only 5 minutes engaged in vigorous activities like running (Nader, 2003; McKenzie, Marshall, Sallis, & Conway, 2000). As noted in chapter 1, it is important that young people spend sufficient time being active, preferably at a level of effort that can provide a health effect. Healthy People 2010 (DHHS, 2000) suggests that students need to be engaged in moderate-to-vigorous physical activity (MVPA) for 50% of the time during physical education class. It is unlikely, though, that this occurs in most physical education classes. A number of instructional strategies, however, can be employed to increase the amount of active time. Some suggestions for increasing physical activity are presented in the sidebar.

Strategies for Increasing Physical Activity Time

1. Efficiency and time management
2. Activity selection
3. Activity organization
4. Equipment availability
5. Instructional organization

Efficiency and Time Management

One of the first areas to address when thinking about organization issues is how best to instruct leaders in effectively coordinating and conducting activity classes. Changing into gym clothes, organizing groups, accounting for attendance, and distributing equipment use up participation time. In addition, transitions from one activity to another may result in unnecessary time lost. From the moment the young person enters the physical activity space, whether in the school gymnasium or the recreation center playground, time is at a premium. So little time is designated for physical activity in today's school curricula that leaders cannot afford to lose precious minutes to inefficient time management. Programs occurring within community settings should also emphasize maximizing activity time. Ways to reduce this time loss should be a focus of any program intervention that seeks to increase physical activity through organized classes.

The online resource for health and physical educators, PE Central (www.pecentral.org), provides an example of how to reduce warm-up and attendance procedures by assigning children numbers or colors that help them direct their own activity at the beginning of class (see sidebar).

Physical Education Will Start at Your Heart

As students enter the gym, they refer to a bulletin board that tells them what they should begin doing immediately. Have them start at PE Numbers. Numbers are located along one wall of the gym. As students enter the gym they proceed to the number 1, where they are instructed to do one of a variety of locomotor skills (walk, skip, crawl, jump, etc.) to get to the opposite side of the gym and then move to the next number (suggested for grades K-3).

Another option is to assign students to begin at various Track Colors. Each color is associated with a station along the track; students perform a variety of warm-up activities as they move around the track. In each of these scenarios, students can proceed through the warm-up stations while the teacher takes attendance, thus eliminating the time normally wasted getting the class organized, taking roll, and starting the first activity (suggested for grades 2-5).

Activity Selection

The type of activities planned and implemented during physical activity programs affects the amount of health-related physical activity children and adolescents are able to accumulate during the program. There are numerous ways to increase class time spent in MVPA to the recommended level of at least 50% of class time if care is taken to choose the proper activities, assess the amount of equipment required, and decrease the size of teams or practice groups.

Different sports and games require different levels of activity from participants. For example, archery is a fun recreational activity, but one that requires little large muscle activity. In comparison, soccer participants are in constant motion, running after the ball and setting up plays. Games and activities can be modified to increase the number of students being physically active at any given time. Softball is a sport commonly offered in middle and high schools, but one in which inactivity is common. Modifications of softball rules could potentially increase MVPA time by allowing fewer foul balls per out, allowing more than one base runner, or requiring students to run the bases before returning to defense.

Offering a variety of activities is important for providing a well-rounded physical activity program for youth. Organized sports do not appeal to all students. Recreation professionals and physical education teachers should think about possibly incorporating other recreational and fitness activities such as hiking, a step class, or in-line skating when planning programs. Providing activities that require moderate or greater exertion levels will positively affect a young person's health.

Activity Organization

A physical activity leader or physical education teacher can employ numerous techniques to maximize the amount of time students spend in activities during the physical activity class. In the CATCH (Coordinated Approach to Child Health) intervention, described in more detail in chapter 4, the amount of time students spent in various levels of physical activity, from sedentary to very active, was assessed before and after classroom teachers and physical education specialists were trained. Increases in physical activity time were noted in classes taught by physical education specialists, primarily because of reductions in time spent standing around (+2.4 minutes). Improvement in classes taught by classroom teachers resulted from reduced sitting (2.2 minutes saved) and increased lesson length (+3.9 minutes) (McKenzie et al., 2001). Professional physical education teachers may not be available for use in most interventions. Thus providing training programs to activity leaders prior to starting an intervention will help to ensure that students receive optimal activity benefits from the program.

Equipment Availability

Traditionally, physical education programs have been inadequately funded, with small or nonexistent budgets for instructional equipment. Having adequate amounts of equipment (balls, hockey sticks, nets, etc.) is essential for maximizing time spent in MVPA. Using only two or three balls for practice in a group of 30 students automatically decreases the number of students who can be active at a given time. Leaders should minimize the amount of time students spend waiting for use of equipment. If the lesson is basketball, the teacher can opt to use volleyballs and soccer balls as well as regulation basketballs to increase the availability of equipment. Even if the equipment is not regulation size, it is more important that all students have as much time as possible to practice passing and dribbling.

Instructional Organization

Using smaller teams or practice groups also will increase the amount of time students spend in MVPA. For example, if students play soccer with teams of three or four players instead of nine, each team member will get more time practicing skills and being active. The Sport Education model (Siedentop, 1994; Siedentop, Hastie, & Vander Mars, 2002) presented in table 3.1 incorporates many of these principles to maximize participation by all students. This model was developed specifically for school curricula, as investigators found that youth were taught activity skills in isolation rather than in the context of sport strategy. The Sport Education model suggests that teams should be kept small and that all students should be given equal play time and an equal opportunity to learn different positions. Students are also encouraged to take on roles other than that of player: they learn how to become referees, managers, organizers, and statisticians. By learning all aspects of a sport, including how to keep score and how to coach a team, youth are presented with a complete sport experience that is greater than if they were merely players (Hastie, 1998). Physical education classes using the Sport Education model have increased time on task as the season progresses. Instead of trying to teach a variety of sports, such classes cover fewer sports, but in greater depth.

A study by Peter Hastie (1998) includes an outline for a curriculum that could be implemented using the Sport Education model (table 3.1). The sport season is broken down into four phases: (1) skill development, (2) preseason scrimmage games, (3) formal competition among teams, and (4) championship playoffs. In the first phase, students are mainly learning the basic skills and rules of the sport. In the second and third phases, teams play scrimmages or actual games. The teacher is head coach during the second phase, but players are also learning their duty roles (e.g., coach, statistician, referee) so that they can take over in the third phase. By the end of the sport season, the instructor's role is that of program director while the students have taken on the roles of coach, referee, scorekeeper, and player. Hastie (1998) found that as the season progressed, children spent less time receiving direct instruction and more time in game play and refereeing roles.

The type of activity selected, the availability of equipment, and the size of teams or practice groups all influence the amount of time students spend being physically active during class. However, you can control your

Table 3.1   Sample Season Outline: Sport Education Model

PHASE	LESSON	FOCUS	TEACHER'S ROLE	STUDENTS' ROLES
1	1	Introduction Rules of game Beginning skills	Class leader	Participant
	2-5	Whole-class skills instruction Team allocation	Class leader Present team lists Discuss roles Discuss fair play	Participant Determine team roles Decide team name
2	6-13	Preseason scrimmages Players learn and practice duty roles	Head coach Referee advisor	Coaches, players Learn duty roles
3	14-25	Formal competition	Program director	Coaches, players Duty team roles
4	26-30	Playoffs Championship game Awards and presentations	Program director Program director Master of ceremonies	Coaches, players Duty team roles Coaches, players Duty team roles

Adapted from Hastie, 1998.

program by thinking about efficient and time-saving practices to engage children and adolescents in more physical activity. By carefully selecting and organizing the activities you focus on, you can provide more MVPA in a limited time.

Designing an Intervention for Skill Development

Increasing the amount of time children and adolescents spend in MVPA during an organized program is not the only way for youth to obtain regular physical activity. Young people accumulate the majority of their physical activity outside of school. Thus, physical activity instructors can encourage increased physical activity outside of the program by giving children and adolescents the skills, knowledge, and motivation needed to adopt and maintain a physically active lifestyle. Social and physical environments can also be altered to provide additional support for physical activity. If the objective of the physical activity program is to produce youth who value activity and engage in it regularly, leaders must understand how to teach such behavior. Children who acquire new skills and learn new information about physical activity are at an advantage with respect to their ability to engage in physical activity successfully. Focusing on the development of motor and behavioral skills, as well as on the dissemination of information about physical activity, is the key technique that influences the time youth spend in physical activity outside of school and in other programs.

Motor Skill Development

Physical activity lessons for children of elementary school ages, whether they are provided through physical education class or another type of intervention, are especially important for developing a child's fundamental locomotor, nonlocomotor (body management), and manipulative skills. Children need time to learn and practice how to jump, throw, skip, hop, catch, and kick; they need experiences in balancing and rolling. Interventions that target this age group should include enhanced instruction for motor skill development.

For the middle school and junior high years, applying motor skills in a variety of game and sport settings is important for youth in transition. It is not necessary, however, that they play structured, competitive games. Young adolescents need variety, which creates interest, and they need occasions to practice skill development (Bell & Darnell, 1994; Sammann, 1998). These opportunities come through program organization and activity selection that provide significant amounts of engagement with the skills of the sport and confidence-building activities. Nonsport activities such as fitness and outdoor recreation activities are effective for use with this age group as well.

As for the high school years, most high school physical education experiences are brief, typically lasting only one year; it is important to offer programs that interest youth at this age. This is the time to direct students' attention toward a lifelong commitment to being active, because interests and preferences are developing. Finding the right activities—those that suit the interests and goals of the individual youth—is critical. Skills developed earlier can be applied to sport, fitness, and leisure activities. Although some students are motivated by competition and enjoy participating in team sports, others may be more interested in noncompetitive activities. Therefore, activity programs should include both competitive sport and lifetime leisure activities such as dance, strength training, jogging, swimming, bicycling, cross-country skiing, walking, and hiking. The LEAP intervention (Lifestyle Education for Activity Project) described in chapter 4 demonstrated an increase in physical activity behavior among high school girls through increased activity time during physical education class and promotion of opportunities outside of class time (Pate et al., 2005).

Behavioral Skill Development

Physical activity leaders should not limit themselves to teaching only motor or sport skills; they also should take on the role of physical health educator. In this capacity, they should be concerned with using concepts that have been shown to influence behavior. Depending on the age of the child or adolescent, a number of different factors appear to influence behavior. As children grow older, their motivations for being active change. At early ages (preschool to early elementary), children move because they love being active, having fun, and playing with their friends. As they progress through elementary school, their awareness of social factors and personal choice grows. As adolescents make the transition from middle to high school, they become more like adults with respect to factors that influence behavior choices. Personal issues such as health (body weight or fitness) may be important, but social influences and competing activities (homework and jobs) are also strong influences on older adolescents.

Many school-based interventions designed to increase physical activity have included a knowledge component as part of the program. Although educating young people about the benefits of physical activity may be important in terms of developing interest, there is no evidence that knowledge itself results in increased participation. In fact, excessive attention to providing information within a class setting is another way in which precious activity time is lost. However, some information is useful and can reinforce activity participation. Important information should be threaded between and into activity segments so as not to detract from the amount of time spent in the activity.

Behavioral determinants for physical activity are factors that have been found to be associated with engagement in physical activity (Heitzler, Martin, Duke, & Huhman, 2006; Kohl and Hobbs, 1998; Sallis, Prochaska, & Taylor, 2000). In a 1998 study, Kohl and Hobbs classified these behavioral influences into three categories: physiological, environmental, and psychosocial factors. Physiological or biological factors that influence physical activity behavior in adolescents include sex, race, and physical health status. In general, more boys than girls are physically active, and youth of color are less active than others. Such differences could be related to body changes during growth for girls or could be due to unexplained social factors in minority youths. Environmental factors include such aspects as how time is spent in physical education classes, availability of sedentary options at home, conduciveness of the weather to active pursuits, and perceptions of neighborhood safety. When environments such as schools, homes, or neighborhoods do not support or facilitate physical activity, young people are less likely to accumulate sufficient amounts of physical activity. Psychosocial factors influencing physical activity include, for example, self-efficacy, beliefs about physical activity, and social influences such as parental and peer support. Perceived self-efficacy has been shown to be strongly correlated with youths' engagement in physical activity because of its link with an individual's motivation and desire to be more physically active. Youth who have a positive attitude toward activity are more likely to engage in it even in the presence of barriers (e.g., weather, access to equipment). Finally, emotional support from both parents and peers correlates with a youth's physically active behaviors.

Physical activity programs should therefore attempt to address some combination of physiological, environmental, and psychosocial factors in order to get youth involved. Chapters 4 through 6 present further information on addressing behavioral factors in the design of a physical activity program. Chapter 4 presents a number of interventions that successfully targeted a variety of behavioral factors in the school setting. Chapter 5 highlights how to engage youth in a community setting, and chapter 6 details approaches to encouraging physical activity in youth in a family-based setting.

SUMMARY

Selection of the setting and the organization of activities are important steps in planning successful physical activity interventions for children and adolescents. Many opportunities exist to design programs that allow youth to accumulate their needed physical activity. Physical education of young people is important in order for them to obtain sufficient physiologic stimulation, develop skills and behaviors, and learn how to seek out physical activity options on their own. Other programmatic avenues such as recreation programs, church programs, or club programs can serve a similar purpose. Taking care to use program time effectively, motivating youth to pursue activities at home or in their community, and providing supportive environments where activity options exist are crucial to a successful intervention design.

Documented Interventions

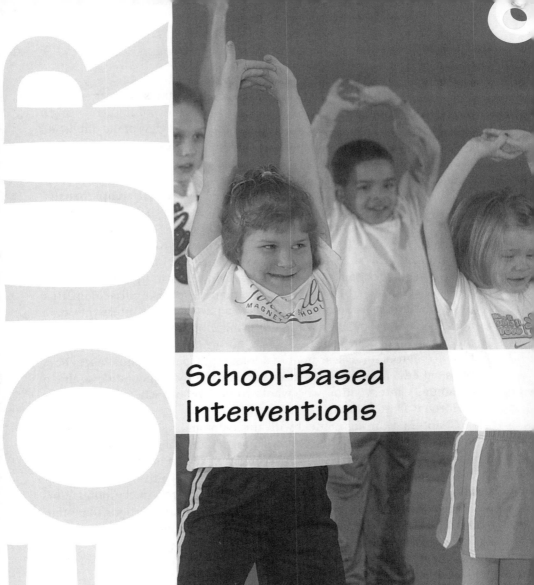

PART two

School-Based Interventions

Learning about theory and considering specific settings are cornerstones in the background research necessary for creating and implementing a new physical activity intervention. Additionally, a review of the published literature is useful for considering what kinds of programs might work in a given setting to reach your goal.

Summaries of published interventions comprise a large portion of part II of this book. Our goal in presenting these is to develop a comprehensive aggregation of interventions and their components that can be used as a resource for program development. With some interventions, such as SPARK (Sports, Play, and Active Recreation for Kids) and NAP SACC (Nutrition and Physical Activity Self-Assessment for Child Care), individuals can acquire training in the program and use it in their own setting. Other programs might have certain elements, such as a curriculum, that program directors can obtain and use as part of a new intervention. In addition, it is important to note that similar approaches can be applied differently depending on the setting. For example, a pedometer might be a useful tool for assessment of adolescents' participation in a school physical education class, or it might be used by someone designing a community intervention who wants to understand where and how far children walk to school.

Chapters 4 through 6 deal with three common settings for physical activity interventions with children and adolescents: schools, the community, and the home. For each setting, we present applicable behavior theory, provide examples of published studies, and introduce issues that might arise in implementing a program. Following this background information on settings and interventions, the third part of this book (chapters 7-10) focuses on tools, ideas, and methods that program leaders can use to design, implement, and assess a physical activity program.

Making the Most of the School Setting

The school setting presents a number of opportunities to intervene with children and adolescents for the purpose of increasing physical activity. Regular, if not daily, physical education is paramount in the effort to increase the moderate-to-vigorous physical activity (MVPA) levels of American youth. An analysis of research-based physical activity interventions showed that physical education interventions were among the more effective approaches (Centers for Disease Control and Prevention

[CDC], 2001). Most young people attend some type of organized physical activity class from elementary through high school. Although there have been decreases in the amount of physical education required in the school curriculum, this organized setting led by professional teachers can be a primary source of physical activity for youth.

The U.S. government's recommendations in Healthy People 2010 (U.S. Department of Health and Human Services, 2000) include numerous goals for physical education in this country, but three main objectives stand out as applicable to youth in a school setting. First, there needs to be an increase in the number of schools that require daily physical education for students. Second, there needs to be an increase in the proportion of youth who participate in daily school physical education. Third, there needs to be an increase in the number of students who spend at least 50% of their physical education classes engaged in physical activity at a level of at least moderate intensity. Baseline information was gathered for high school (9th-12th grade) age adolescents, and target percentages were set for these three objectives. Both are presented in table 4.1, adapted from Healthy People 2010 (http://healthypeople.gov).

It is clear that an imperative exists for health and educational professionals to educate children and youth about physical activity behaviors. Before we present examples of published intervention studies, it is necessary to examine the theoretical constructs that influence physical activity behavior, as different constructs must be targeted by different programs.

Table 4.1 Healthy People 2010 Objectives for High School Physical Education

SECTION	OBJECTIVE	1994 BASELINE	2010 TARGET
22-8	Increase the number of the nation's public and private schools that require daily physical education for all students	2%	5%
22-9	Increase the proportion of adolescents who participate in daily school physical education	29%	50%
22-10	Increase the proportion of adolescents who spend at least 50% of school physical education class time being physically active	38%	50%

Adapted from Healthy People 2010.

Using Behavior Theory in School-Based Interventions

As discussed in chapter 2, experts organize the influences on physical activity into different levels, providing what is known as an ecological model, and recommend using this multilevel approach to understand and promote physical activity. Because there are many influences on physical activity in youth, interventions or programs that target several of them simultaneously are more likely to be effective in changing behavior than programs that target only one influence. Programs directed at a single influence are often implemented through instructional components, such as health education and physical education, and include activities or instruction designed to increase physical activity self-efficacy; change beliefs, attitudes, or knowledge related to physical activity; increase intentions to be physically active; increase skills to adopt and maintain a physically active lifestyle; and develop activity- and sport-specific skills (Stone, McKenzie, Welk, & Booth, 1998).

Programs that target different ecological levels, however, might pair instruction with social support, organizational change, or collaboration with the community. Interpersonal approaches might be implemented as program components that involve peers and parents as positive influences and develop social support for physical activity. Organizational approaches involve changes to the school organization. For example, the school provides access to fun opportunities and has policies that support physical activities such as enrollment in a daily physical education class. The school might provide training to teachers and staff to ensure that they are skilled at engaging youth in enjoyable physical activity. Community and environmental approaches involve collaboration between the school and community agencies to increase the availability of physical activity programs, access to facilities, and opportunities in the community. Those approaches also include developing physical activity events coordinated by both the school and the community and advocating changes in the environment that will increase accessibility to safe physical activity opportunities for all youth.

In table 4.2, we present a way of organizing constructs from social cognitive theory and applying them to intervention programs that could be administered in a school setting. By identifying constructs at multiple levels, you increase the chance that your program will be successful in changing physical activity behavior.

Table 4.2 Ecological Approach to Organizing Theory Constructs in School Settings

INFLUENCES ON BEHAVIOR	APPLICATION FOR INTERVENTIONS
Individual	
• Perceived self-efficacy • Expectations (including perceived benefits and barriers) • Intention to be physically active • Behavioral skills • Behavioral capability	• Physical education instruction is modified to increase enjoyment of physical activity. • Physical activity outside of physical education is promoted. • Health education instruction is designed to develop behavioral skills for physical activity such as goal setting, overcoming barriers, and seeking support.
Interpersonal	
• Social environment from social cognitive theory (including modeling and observational learning) • Social support/Social network • Social influence approaches	• Changing physical education so that students can interact socially while being physically active, such as working in pairs. • Incorporating homework that involves family in activities.
Organizational	
• Organizational change • Policies	• School policy for daily physical education. • Increase the amount of physical education required, such as from once to twice per week. • School policy requires mandatory recess period for early elementary grades.
Community	
• Interorganizational relations • Community development • Advocacy approaches	• School and recreation agency collaborate to provide after-school physical activity programs. • Neighborhood coalition is formed to get sidewalks built so children can walk to school.

In order to promote physical activity at school, one can design a variety of different interventions. The four main types that are found in published literature include quality physical education programs, physical education–only interventions, physical activity in the classroom, and comprehensive or coordinated interventions. These are defined in

Table 4.3   Types of Physical Activity School Intervention Programs

TYPE	DEFINITION
Quality physical education programs	Enhancements of existing physical education programs
Physical education–only interventions	Interventions that increase the amount or enjoyment of physical education classes
Physical activity in the classroom	Interventions that add an activity component to the academic classroom
Comprehensive or coordinated interventions	Interventions that use a number of school components to increase physical activity in youth

table 4.3 and are presented in further detail in the following sections, along with examples of published interventions that have targeted youth in the school setting.

Developing Quality Physical Education Programs

Many groups have highlighted the need for increased physical activity among America's youth, including increasing both the quantity and quality of physical education classes. Healthy People 2010 includes specific objectives targeted at physical education, while the National Association for Sport and Physical Education (NASPE) defines standards for physical education and for what a physically educated person should be able to accomplish. In 2000, the Secretary of Health and Human Services and the Secretary of Education presented a joint recommendation to describe and emphasize the importance of quality physical education. Table 4.4 includes both the joint statement and the NASPE guidelines.

Many national publications have recognized the potential for physical education programs to increase the physical activity levels of children and adolescents. Physical education not only provides an opportunity for increased physical activity as a result of class participation, it also gives youth an opportunity to learn physical and behavioral skills that they can use outside of school to remain physically active. These lifetime benefits are well documented in "Guidelines for School and Community Programs to Promote Lifelong Physical Activity Among Young People," a research-based publication by the Centers for Disease Control and

Table 4.4 Recommendations for Physical Education

THE PHYSICALLY EDUCATED PERSON	QUALITY PHYSICAL EDUCATION
1. Demonstrates competency in many movement forms and proficiency in a few movement forms. 2. Applies involvement concepts and principles to the learning and development of motor skills. 3. Exhibits a physically active lifestyle. 4. Achieves and maintains a health-enhancing level of physical fitness. 5. Demonstrates responsible personal and social behavior in physical activity settings. 6. Demonstrates understanding of and respect for differences among people in physical activity settings. 7. Understands that physical activity provides opportunities for enjoyment, challenge, self-expression, and social interaction. Source: National Association for Sport and Physical Education (1995).	1. Provides intense instruction in motor and self-management skills needed to enjoy a variety of physical activities. 2. Keeps students active for most of the class period. 3. Builds students' confidence in their physical abilities. 4. Influences moral development by providing students with opportunities to assume leadership, cooperate with others, and accept responsibility for their own behavior. 5. Is fun! Source: U.S. Department of Health and Human Services and U.S. Department of Education (2000).

Prevention (CDC, 1997). This publication emphasizes that physical education programs can substantially contribute to youth physical activity, both through direct provision of time to engage in MVPA and through educational and promotional activities that give students the motor skills, physical fitness, and behavioral skills to seek out and engage in physical activity for a lifetime.

CDC Recommendation for Physical Education

Implement physical education curricula and instruction that emphasize enjoyable participation in physical activity and that help students develop the knowledge, attitudes, motor skills, behavioral skills, and confidence needed to adopt and maintain physically active lifestyles (CDC, 1997).

The objectives set out by Healthy People 2010, and the recommendations of NASPE and the Secretaries of Health and Human Services and

Education, can be summarized into two broad categories: those that seek to increase physical activity in schools, and those that seek to encourage physical activity outside of school. It is difficult for children and adolescents to meet the recommended levels of physical activity through physical education classes alone. Quality physical education programs can maximize the amount of time children are physically active at school and encourage them to continue physical activity outside of school.

Evaluating Physical Education Interventions

Just a few physical education–only interventions have been evaluated for their effectiveness in increasing the physical activity behavior of children or adolescents. Most school-based interventions have included a physical education component along with other components such as health education. Examples of these interventions are discussed in the following sections and are presented for quick reference in table 4.5 at the end of the chapter.

SPARK: Sports, Play, and Active Recreation for Kids

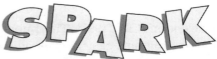

SPARK (Sallis et al., 1997) included 10 health-related activity units and nine sport units and taught self-management skills (self-monitor-ing, goal setting, stimulus control, self-reinforcement, self-instruction, and problem solving). A major emphasis in the SPARK curriculum was to improve teacher efficiency and to increase the amount of MVPA obtained during class time. Enjoyment was also emphasized.

SPARK was originally evaluated with classes of fourth- and fifth-grade students to test the effectiveness of its curriculum, led by physical education specialists or trained classroom teachers, as compared to traditional physical education programs. The program was designed to be taught three days per week for 30 minutes, although adherence varied greatly. Traditional PE classes provided only 18 minutes of MVPA per week, whereas classroom teachers and physical education specialists using SPARK provided 33 and 40 minutes of MVPA, respectively. Follow-up studies testing institutionalization of concepts and methods have demonstrated sustainability. Additionally, significant increases were obtained in fitness among girls and in sport skills (such as throwing, catching, and kicking) among all youth. Since its inception, SPARK has evolved to include programs for a variety of age groups (pre-K, K-2, grades 3-6, middle school, high school, and after school). More information about the SPARK curriculum can be found on the program's Web site (www. sparkpe.org) or via e-mail (spark@sparkpe.org).

M-SPAN: Middle School Physical Activity and Nutrition

M-SPAN was an intervention in which the major component was an enhanced physical education program (McKenzie et al., 2004). This project was the first of its kind to target middle school students. The M-SPAN intervention included curricular materials, staff development, and on-site follow-up. Teacher training focused on awareness of the need for active and health-related physical education programs, design and implementation of an active curriculum, improvements in classroom management and organizational strategies for activity, and ongoing teacher support. After a two-year implementation period, MVPA in physical education class increased by 18%, or approximately 3 minutes per lesson. Boys responded better to this approach than girls, but overall M-SPAN shows much promise for increasing physical activity during physical education class. Further information about M-SPAN can be found online (www. sparkpe.org/programMiddlePE.jsp).

South Australia Daily Physical Education Study

Increasing the scheduled time for physical education classes can be an effective way to add more physical activity to the lives of youth; however, school districts need evidence that the effort is worthy of the cost required to add more physical education to the curriculum. Three approaches to physical education were compared in the South Australia study by Dwyer and colleagues (1983). A traditional 30-minute physical education class scheduled three times per week was compared to either a skills training approach or a fitness training approach, both offered daily for 75 minutes. Intensity was emphasized in the fitness class. After 14 weeks, the fitness group showed a significant increase in aerobic fitness and decrease in body fat skinfold measurements compared to the other two groups. There was no evidence of loss of academic performance based on math and reading tests in spite of the loss of formal teaching time.

Adding Physical Activity to the Classroom

As noted earlier, increasing the amount of time appropriated for physical education class and making the physical education class a source of MVPA can result in measurable increases in the time children and adolescents spend in physical activity. However, other subjects like language arts, math, and science can incorporate physical activity time or promote an interest in physical activity through the lesson plan. In science class, for example, a teacher might assign students to play "Energy Tag" (see sidebar), an activity suggested on the PE Central Web site to teach elementary school students about how blood carries oxygen and elevate their heart rates through physical activity.

Energy Tag

- The science teacher sets up an obstacle course for students that represents the path that blood takes to carry oxygen from the lungs to the heart and to the body (muscles) to create energy.
- A series of tunnels and hurdles are set up to represent different points in the pathway. For example, one tunnel can be labeled "Right Atrium—walk or crawl," followed by a tunnel labeled "Tricuspid Valve to Right Ventricle—walk or crawl."
- Four to five students are designated "taggers."
- The rest of the students travel through the obstacle course collecting red flags representing oxygen in the lungs, and the "taggers," representing muscles, try to grab these flags as the students pass through the portion of the course representing the body.

Source: PE Central

Programs that have been specifically designed to help teachers improve the level of physical activity within their classrooms include Take 10!, PLAY, and JumpSTART.

Take 10!

TAKE 10! is a classroom-based physical activity program for elementary schools. To reinforce learning objectives and promote health, TAKE 10! integrates physical activity and nutrition concepts with grade-specific academic lessons in language arts, math, social studies, science, nutrition, health, 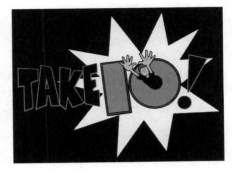 and character education. For instance, movement of the arms can be integrated into math classes by teaching students to tell time using their own bodies to model the face and hands of a clock, and various physical activities can be incorporated into a traditional spelling lesson by encouraging children to jump, do a pushup, or jog in place while calling out the letters. The 10-minute moderate-to-vigorous physical activities can replace a seated classroom lesson and require no special equipment or training for teachers. Activities include a cool-down period to transition students back to their seats. During the cool-down period, grade-specific nutrition or health questions can be reviewed with students. Materials, including activity cards, academically linked worksheets, tracking posters and stickers, are available for elementary school teachers through the Take 10! Web site at www.take10.net.

An intervention that used Take 10! in addition to other classroom-based instructional modules received enthusiastic endorsement from teachers for creating 10 minutes of active instructional time on a daily basis. Physical activity levels of the children increased, and a majority of teachers (75%) were able to use the materials on most days of the week (Stewart, Dennison, Kohl, & Doyle, 2004). Take 10! has been employed by schools to supplement the amount of physical activity obtained by children during the school day (Plescia, Young, & Ritzman, 2005).

PLAY: Promoting Lifetime Activity for Youth

A similar approach was employed by researchers to meet the physical activity recommendations of the Arizona Department of Education Comprehensive Health Education Standards. PLAY was designed as a supplement to physical education classes with the goal of increased MVPA levels and improved active lifestyle habits. This intervention was designed for implementation by classroom teachers and was tested with fourth-, fifth-, and sixth-grade students (Ernst & Pangrazi, 1999). Fifteen-minute activity breaks were incorporated into each school day by teachers and were supplemented by weekly goals of 30 minutes of accumulated activity at least five days per week. The PLAY intervention was successful in increasing physical activity levels for both boys and girls in this age group.

JumpSTART

JumpSTART was developed for the National Recreation and Park Association in order to promote a healthy, active lifestyle for children through incorporation of physical activity and nutritional information into the school curriculum. Targeted at grades

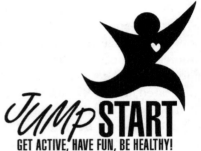

3 through 5, JumpSTART includes a variety of activities that can help teachers instill in children the importance of healthy eating and physical activity. This program includes 10 specific suggestions for math, science, social studies, and language arts classes. In language arts, for example, teachers might take students on a walk in a park or on the school grounds while encouraging them to observe and describe the natural world in the way a poet would. Other suggestions can be found on the JumpSTART Web site (www.nhlbi.nih.gov/health/prof/heart/other/jumpstrt.htm). In addition to school-based activities, JumpSTART provides materials that children can share with their parents.

Promoting Physical Activity With Comprehensive and Coordinated Interventions

Some physical activity interventions include, in addition to physical education, other aspects of the school health program, which allows the intervention to leverage a number of components to increase physical activity behavior or to focus on a health outcome such as enhanced cardiovascular health or the prevention of obesity. School-based programs that have a broader focus than just physical education are organized as either comprehensive or coordinated intervention programs.

Comprehensive programs that promote physical activity in school settings involve such classroom components as physical education and health education and such environmental components as school food service and school policies that affect physical activity. These programs might focus on health behaviors like physical activity, dietary behavior, and tobacco use, or they might focus on health outcomes influenced by physical activity such as obesity, serum cholesterol, and other cardiovascular risk factors.

Coordinated programs in school settings are often comprehensive in that they might include both instructional and policy changes to encourage youth to be more physically active. The greater emphasis in these programs, however, is on coordination at the school level. A coordinated program will have a committee or team that serves as a coordinating body and is made up of teachers, school officials, parents, and other community members. Figure 4.1 illustrates the CDC's Coordinated School

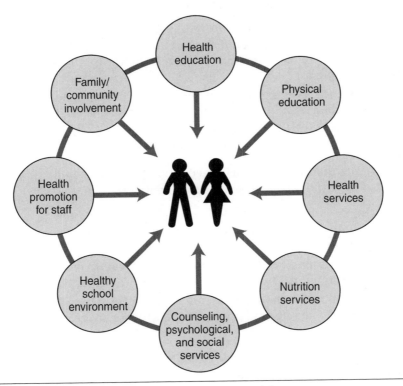

Figure 4.1 Coordinated School Health Program model.

Adapted from the Centers for Disease Control and Prevention (CDC).

Health Program model. This model is composed of eight interactive components and illustrates the importance of involving educators, families, communities, religious organizations, and medical professionals in addressing the country's health problems. Further explanation of each of the eight components can be found on the CDC's Web site (www.cdc.gov/HealthyYouth/CSHP/).

An important requirement of such a program is that the coordinating team be recognized as the official coordinating body for the work of these eight components (Allensworth, Lawson, Nicholson, & Wyche, 1997). Many schools have some or all of these elements in place, but what makes the program coordinated is the existence of positive working relationships among the various groups. Success is enhanced by the leadership and negotiation skills of the coordinating team.

There are several advantages of comprehensive and coordinated programs for promoting physical activity:

- They include different levels of impact (personal, social, and environmental) that are recommended for promoting physical activity and are more likely to create change in behavior and in the school environment.
- They entail working with existing school resources and programs, rather than creating new structures that must be added.
- They provide the opportunity for reinforcement of health messages through multiple approaches and channels.

Programs that are developed in collaboration with community agencies also have the following potential advantages:

- Schools and community agencies can work together to achieve common goals that individual organizations could not achieve working alone.
- Such programs can help schools and communities make the best use of limited resources.
- They can help school and community collaborators develop their capacity to identify and solve problems that might arise in the future (see Fetro, 1998).

The following sections provide examples of comprehensive and coordinated programs that were successful in promoting physical activity and other healthy behaviors, organized by grade level (elementary, middle, and high schools).

Elementary School Programs

The elementary school level programs that we discuss here are CATCH—Coordinated Approach to Child Health; CHIC—Cardiovascular Health in Children; Go for Health; Pathways; and Eat Well and Keep Moving.

CATCH: Coordinated Approach to Child Health

CATCH, an intervention based on social cognitive theory and organizational change theory, was originally targeted at third-, fourth-, and fifth-grade children under the name Child and Adolescent Trial for Cardiovascular Health. The intervention focused on modifications in physical education classes, changes in school lunches, and fostering increased family involvement. CATCH was designed to pro-

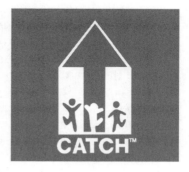

mote more healthful eating by decreasing fat and salt in children's diets, increase physical activity, and prevent tobacco use in order to have a positive influence on cholesterol, blood pressure, and physical fitness. School curricula focused on health behaviors, which were to be reinforced by parents through parental involvement programs. Finally, the behavior changes were supported by changes in the school environment: Cafeterias served lower-fat foods, physical education teachers had children participate in MVPA for at least 50% of class time, and schoolwide anti-tobacco literature was displayed (Luepker et al., 1996). CATCH programs were experimentally implemented in 56 schools in four states.

After three years, data were assessed on food service, classroom activities, physical education, and home programs. High levels of participation continued throughout this time, and children who participated in CATCH were found to be less likely to consume high-fat foods and were more likely to be physically active outside of school (Perry et al., 1997). This multilevel intervention has thus been shown to help promote exercising and healthy eating among elementary school children. The CATCH program is now known as the Coordinated Approach to Child Health because of its promotion from a research trial to a continuing and successful program. More information can be found on the program's Web site (www.catchinfo.org).

CHIC: Cardiovascular Health in Children

The CHIC study, based on social cognitive theory, targeted third- and fourth-grade children in rural 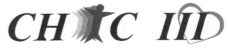 North Carolina through both classroom and physical education components (Harrell et al., 1996). The classroom curriculum, a condensed version of the American Heart Association curriculum available at the time (1990-1991), was delivered to all students for eight weeks by either the regular classroom teacher or a certified physical education teacher. In addition, a certified physical education teacher taught the physical education curriculum for three sessions per week during the eight weeks of the program. Two interventions were actually staged: one for all third and fourth graders, and one for a risk-based population that was split into small groups of six to eight children. The latter population was composed of children whose parents reported a family history of cardiovascular disease (e.g., heart attack, high blood pressure, stroke). The large-group intervention was actually more successful than the small-group intervention in reducing body fat, improving aerobic fitness through physical activity, and increasing health knowledge among the children. In addition, the large-group intervention was less costly and easier to implement than the more individualized program. For more information about past and ongoing CHIC studies, see the program's Web site (www.unc.edu/depts/chic/).

Go for Health

Go for Health, based on organizational change and social cognitive theories, sought to increase healthful eating and physical activity among third- and fourth-grade students (Parcel, Simons-Morton, O'Hara, Baranowski, & Wilson, 1989). The program worked to reduce sodium, fat, and saturated fat in school lunches; to increase the amount of time children were physically active in physical education through a new curriculum; and to develop students' knowledge, skills, behavioral capability, confidence, and positive expectations related to physical activity through health instruction. The physical education curriculum consisted of two semester-long units, six to eight weeks each, that emphasized having fun while being physically active. The health education curriculum consisted of two four-week modules on healthy eating and one six-week module about physical activity. The project dietitian worked with school cafeteria staff to modify purchasing, menu planning, recipe development, and food preparation. Physical education and health education teachers were trained to implement the curricula. Results from the Go for Health program indicate positive outcomes for self-efficacy in that children felt more confident about their ability to change their behavior and understand future outcomes. In addition to a decline in salt intake, participation in aerobic physical activity increased owing to the positive influence of the health education curriculum.

Pathways

Based on social cognitive theory, Pathways targeted rural American Indian children in third, fourth, and fifth grades from 41 schools in seven American Indian Nations (Caballero et al., 2003). The intervention emphasized developing a culturally appropriate curriculum that promoted healthful eating behaviors with an aim of preventing obesity and other health problems. In addition, the Pathways program had family, food service, and physical activity components. The family component, geared toward increasing family support and involvement, included family fun night, family events and workshops, year-end celebration events, and family information sheets. The food service component was devised to work with existing cafeteria services in order to design and serve meals that were lower in fat. It included nutrient and behavioral guidelines, support materials and activities, training sessions for food service staff, and kitchen visits. The physical activity components, designed to increase in-school physical activity opportunities, included SPARK physical education, exercise breaks, American Indian games, and an increase in recess time per week. The results of this program indicate that children gained knowledge about healthy behaviors, that training school food service professionals resulted in significant changes in regard to the fat content of food served in schools, and that there was a positive trend in the amount of physical activity added to the school day. More information on this intervention can be found on the Pathways Web site (http://hsc.unm.edu/pathways/).

Eat Well and Keep Moving

Based on social cognitive theory, social marketing, and behavior choice theory, Eat Well and Keep Moving was designed by Harvard researchers to promote the physical and nutritional education of 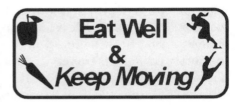 fourth- and fifth-grade students in Baltimore (Gortmaker, Cheung, et al., 1999). The specific goals were to get students to eat more fruits and vegetables and less fat, and to be more physically active and less inactive. The intervention had six interlinked components: classroom education, food service, physical education, staff wellness, parental involvement, and schoolwide promotional campaigns that were designed both to create a supportive learning environment and to work with existing school resources and curricula. The physical education component reinforced messages received in the classroom by using lesson plans that integrated physical activity and nutrition. Results of the study (Gortmaker, Peterson, et al., 1999) indicated that children's diets improved, particularly with regard to an increase in vitamin C and consumption of fruits and vegetables, because the children were able to make changes in their own behavior. Physical activities were not significantly improved over the course of the study; however, all the schools targeted had little physical education time and few after-school programs, which likely contributed to the limitations of increasing physical activity. More information about this intervention can be found on the project's Web site (www.hsph. harvard.edu/prc/proj_eat.html).

Middle School Programs

The middle school level programs that we discuss here are Planet Health and Trial of Activity in Adolescent Girls (TAAG).

Planet Health

Based on social cognitive theory and behavioral choice theory, the Planet Health intervention targeted the prevention of obesity in children in sixth, seventh, and eighth grade in five different Massachusetts public schools (Gortmaker, Peterson, et al., 1999). The intervention was an interdisciplinary curriculum that focused on improving the health and well-being of students in terms of physical activity and nutrition. Adolescents were encouraged to consume more fruits and vegetables while changing their dietary habits, and they were encouraged to limit their television viewing in order to accommodate more physical activity each day. In order to accomplish this, Planet Health wove information about healthy eating and activity behaviors into math, science, language arts, social studies, and physical education for all students, not just those at risk for obesity. These materials, designed to integrate with the existing public school curriculum, included 32 classroom lessons and 30 brief lessons in physical education. At the end of the two-year intervention period, obesity prevalence declined 3.3% for girls and 1.5% for boys. In addition, the researchers noted a decrease in time spent watching television, as well as an increase in fruit and vegetable consumption. More information about Planet Health can be found on the program's Web site (www.hsph.harvard.edu/prc/proj_planet.html).

TAAG: Trial of Activity for Adolescent Girls

TAAG is a national study involving middle schools in six different areas of the country (Young et al., 2006; Gittelsohn et al., 2006). It promotes physical activity in middle school, with the goal of forestalling the downward trend 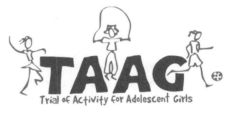 often seen in physical activity levels among girls in this age group. TAAG has four primary components: physical education, health education with activity challenges, promotion, and programs for physical activity. The health and physical education components are classroom based; the promotion component includes a variety of promotional and media activities to encourage and support physical activity; and the programs for physical activity are designed to link girls to physical activity opportunities in the community, particularly after school. More information can be found on the TAAG Web site (www.cscc.unc.edu/taag/).

High School Programs

The two high school level programs we discuss here are New Moves and Lifestyle Education for Activity Project (LEAP).

New Moves

New Moves was designed as an obesity prevention program for high school girls that could be implemented so as to avoid stigmatizing overweight girls and to help them avoid the risk of unhealthy weight loss practices by increasing their feelings of self-efficacy and enjoyment of activities (Neumark-Sztainer, Story, Hannan, & Rex, 2003). Based on social cognitive theory, this program addressed environmental, personal, and behavioral elements in the girls' lives through alternative physical education and information sessions. As a part of physical education, participants were exposed to a variety of community opportunities in physical activity. The physical activity sessions promoted lifelong physical activities for girls of different sizes, shapes, and skill levels within a supportive and noncompetitive environment. Nutrition sessions focused on increasing fruit and vegetable intake while decreasing consumption of foods high in fat and sugar. Girls were encouraged to avoid dieting. The social support sessions focused on increasing self-image and awareness of media messages about body weight, on learning healthful ways to manage stress, and on providing support for change.

New Moves was implemented by school staff in conjunction with research team members. The physical education component was taught by a school physical education teacher; social support sessions were led by either a school counselor or a member of the New Moves research team; the nutrition component was taught by a member of the New Moves research team who was a registered dietitian. By introducing psychological support networks and nutrition information, New Moves helped students increase their physical activity, improve their dietary habits, and enhance their self-image. Positive changes in behavior were seen in the intervention group, including increased time devoted to physical activity each week and an increase in consumption of healthy foods like fruits and vegetables. Parental and peer support increased during and after the study, demonstrating a change in social support. In addition, girls in the intervention were found to have higher rates of self-acceptance, self-worth, and general acceptance of their physical appearance (Neumark-Sztainer et al., 2003, p. 48). Parents and school leaders all expressed support for the continuation of the program.

LEAP: Lifestyle Education for Activity Project

LEAP was a physical activity promotion intervention targeting high school girls using six of the eight components of the Coordinated School Health Program (figure 4.1) to promote activity: physical education, health education, health services, faculty/ 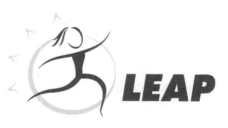 staff wellness, family and community involvement, and healthy school environment (Pate et al., 2005). LEAP worked with school teachers and staff to modify the existing physical education curriculum in order to make it more attractive to girls and ensure that participants were physically active during class. Some of these changes included providing girls-only physical education, providing girls a choice in activities, encouraging appropriate social interaction in physical education class, focusing on lifelong physical activity, including noncompetitive activities in physical education, and linking girls to physical activity opportunities in the community. The health education component, which was implemented in a variety of classes including health, physical education, and science, was designed to provide girls with the behavioral skills to become and remain physically active. In the health services component, the school nurse was involved in promoting physical activity, and in the family and community involvement component, a variety of activities promoted linkages to physical activity outside of school. Finally, the healthy school environment component involved the development of the LEAP team, a coordinating committee for promoting physical activity in the school. Results indicate that LEAP was successful in increasing physical activity in intervention schools (Pate et al., 2005).

Working Effectively With Schools

In chapter 7 we discuss the basic elements for physical activity program planning, including the target group for the program, cooperating professionals (change agents), the type of physical activity behavior to be changed, and where and when the program will take place. The summary table on page 84 shows these basic elements, as well as program components, for the interventions described in the previous sections.

Based on the theoretical orientation and published studies we have described, it is obvious that many comprehensive school-based programs involve change at individual, interpersonal, and organizational levels. There is increasing emphasis on including community- or environmental-level influences, particularly school and community agency collaboration that will provide physical activity opportunities for youth. For example, a school and a local recreation commission can work together to provide after-school physical activity programs for students. The final section of this chapter deals with issues you might encounter in collaborating with schools.

If you are an outside group or community agency and wish to target your intervention at the school setting, collaboration between the school and the outside organization rests on four key elements: understanding the school system, gaining entrance into the school system, working together effectively, and maintaining the relationship.

- **Understanding the system.** Professionals entering a school as outsiders must keep in mind that the priority of the school is education for its students, and one of its biggest concerns is the well-being of the students and the adults who work with them. Anything that is perceived as a threat to the school's priorities or to students and school employees will not be welcomed into the school. Ideally, intervention program personnel need to explain clearly how their activities will further the school's mission. At the very least, they must show that what they are proposing will not take away from what the school believes is important. Providing this assurance to the school will require more than a single contact or the delivery of a brochure.

- **Gaining entrance.** In working with schools, interested parties must allow plenty of time to make the appropriate contacts, develop relationships, and deliver their program. Most schools already have established procedures for outsiders (e.g., agencies, groups, parents) to gain appropriate entry. In order to implement interventions, program directors will also be required to go through the appropriate approval process, regardless of the scope of the project. Most schools require district-level approval in addition to school-level approval. It will be important to identify specific individuals at these levels who can facilitate requests for entry. Telephone contacts should be followed up with written confirmation. Data collection must follow school or district procedures, as well as those required by the interested outside agency.

- **Working together.** Professional etiquette should be observed in all dealings with school employees, including contact with the students. Impediments to accessibility and other challenges must be met with flexibility. Program staff must be willing to negotiate and compromise when needed, with respect for the school and its students and staff. Outsiders must always work with the school to protect the privacy of individuals, both adults and children, and to minimize disruption to the school day. You also must remember to express appreciation to administrators, staff, teachers, and students at every appropriate opportunity. Each of the reasons an outside professional has for seeking entry into a school might encompass different expectations concerning the role of the school and the role of the outside group. Program directors must ensure that all parties understand the purposes of the collaboration as well as role expectations and levels of commitment.

- **Maintaining relationships.** Relationships are built on positive interpersonal contact. To maintain an effective relationship with the school, outsiders must always show respect. To develop trust, they should behave in a trustworthy manner that demonstrates genuine concern for the school, the school's mission, and the students' education and well-being. Relationships are sustained over time with the development of common goals and effective communication.

SUMMARY

Many examples of school-based programs to promote physical activity in children and adolescents have been published. Many programs classified as comprehensive have been published, but several physical education–only studies have also been conducted. The number and type of components included in these programs relate to the goals and objectives of the program. For example, programs that focus on body weight-related outcomes might have physical activity and food service components. All programs included physical education. Most of the programs were delivered in the school by local personnel serving as change agents who had been trained by the research staff. Generally, the programs had some flexibility built into them to accommodate variations among schools. For example, health education content and skills might be delivered within a variety of subjects since there is much variation in health education provided by schools. Most of the programs reviewed have had positive effects on physical activity in school, especially within physical education. However, fewer school-based programs have had a significant effect on physical activity outside of school.

Experts recommend developing school-based programs that build on current successes and that have a greater focus on promoting out-of-school physical activity. The ecological model, in characterizing approaches to theory that can be useful for targeting children and adolescents in a school setting, can help planners create and implement physical activity programs. Planners can also benefit from examples of published interventions and from information about their designs and results, and outside agents who want to work with schools need to understand how to collaborate effectively with the school.

Summary of Basic Elements for School-Based Programs

INTER-VENTION	TARGET	CHANGE AGENTS	PROGRAM COMPONENTS	PHYSICAL ACTIVITY BEHAVIOR
Elementary school				
CATCH	Grades K-5	Physical education teachers, cafeteria workers	Curricula, physical education, lunch, family, policy	MVPA in physical education and out of school
CHIC	Grades 3-4	Classroom teachers, physical education teachers	Health curriculum, physical education	Physical activity and fitness
Eat Well and Keep Moving	Grades 4-5	Classroom teachers, physical education teachers, food service staff	Classroom education, physical education, food services, staff wellness, parent involvement, and promotional campaign	Increased physical activity
Go for Health	Grades 3-4	Classroom teachers, physical education teachers, food service staff	Physical education curriculum, health education curriculum, food service	MVPA in physical education, out-of-school physical activity
Pathways	American Indian children, grades 3-5	Classroom teachers, physical education teachers, food service staff	Physical activity, family, food service	Physical activity

INTER-VENTION	TARGET	CHANGE AGENTS	PROGRAM COMPONENTS	PHYSICAL ACTIVITY BEHAVIOR
Elementary school (continued)				
PLAY	Grades 4-6	Classroom teachers	15 minutes of activity time	Increased physical activity
South Australia Daily Physical Education Study	Grade 5	Physical education teachers	75 minutes of fitness-based physical education every day	Increased fitness
Middle school				
Take 10!	Grades K-5, 6-8	Classroom teachers	10 minutes of activity time	Increased physical activity
M-SPAN	Middle school grades 6-8	Physical education teachers	Physical education curriculum	MVPA in physical education
Planet Health	Grades 6-7	Classroom teachers in math, science, language arts, social studies, and physical education teachers	Classroom and physical education	MVPA
TAAG	Grades 6-8	Classroom teachers, physical education teachers, community agency staff	Classroom, physical education, promotion, and programs with community agencies	MVPA
High school				
New Moves	Females in high school	Classroom teachers, guidance counselors	Classroom education, physical education, social support	Physical activity
LEAP	Females in high school	Physical education teachers, classroom teachers, and school staff	Physical education, health education, health promotion for staff, health services, family-community involvement, and healthy environment	MVPA in physical education and out of school

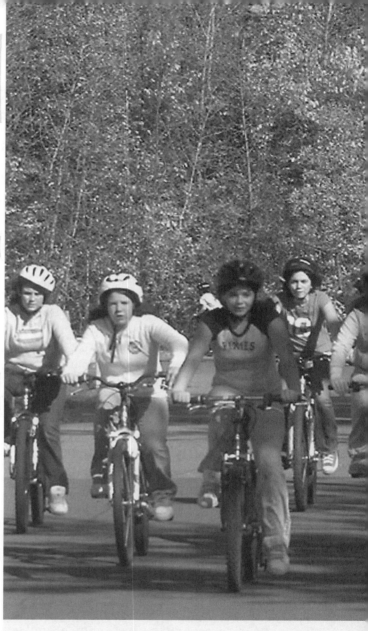

FIVE

Community Interventions

Children and adolescents get most of their physical activity after school. They participate in sport programs, take dance or karate lessons, or just spend time riding bikes and playing with friends. On weekends and in the summers, young people are free to pursue their interests most of the day. Although many youth participate in community sports and recreation, for others, these are times of missed opportunities for physical activity (Sturm, 2005). For inactive young people, the hours between school and bedtime are time to watch TV or videos, play video games, use the computer, or talk on the telephone. Although the nonschool period has much potential for physical activity interventions, few formal interventions have been developed to address youth who are inactive outside of the school setting. As alarm grows over the increased levels of obesity in our society and the relationship of physical inactivity to this problem, employing numerous community settings and these rich time opportunities for intervention might be very useful.

Chapter 4 highlighted interventions that take place during the school day. In this chapter, we focus on community interventions in a variety of neighborhood settings as well as after-school interventions at school. Although home-based and health care interventions are also considered community programs, these will be addressed in chapter 6.

Making the Most of the Community Setting

In intervention development, a community is any group of individuals connected by some aspect of their lives, including geography (neighborhood or housing development), social interaction (religious affiliation or club membership), or shared identity (ethnic group) (Pate et al., 2000). Community physical activity settings might include the following:

- Schools (during and after school)
- Religious institutions (e.g., church youth groups)
- Social and fraternal organizations (e.g., Boy Scouts)
- Neighborhood groups (e.g., housing developments or community clubhouses)
- Community-based organizations (e.g., Boys & Girls Clubs or YMCA)
- Streets, parks, and greenways (around a specific neighborhood)

- Clinical settings (e.g., physician's office or health department clinic)
- Media (e.g., TV, magazines, or billboards)

Many community intervention programs have been developed in appropriate settings to target specific communities, such as Latino youth in a soccer league or African American girls living in public housing.

Unlike interventions that take place at school, community interventions take place in programs that children and adolescents are not required to attend. Youth can choose to attend or not attend, can come late and leave early, or can drop out entirely. Young people might have more motivation for physical activity in a community-based program than in school because they chose to attend it. In addition, community settings might be able to provide a greater variety of physical activity opportunities compared to those available at school because they are not constrained by geography. Other beneficial aspects of community-based physical activity programs include opportunities to make physical activity the social norm, or the "thing to do." Included in community programs are important adults like coaches, family members, or church leaders. Community programs or initiatives might also institute permanent changes in the physical environment, such as the development of a playground or a walking trail or the development of policies that provide greater access to physical activity programs or spaces (e.g., opening school gyms during the evening for community use).

Using Behavior Theory in Community Interventions

Community-based, youth-oriented physical activity programs should focus not only on the individual child, but also on other components of the environment that affect young people's physical activity. These include the social setting, the physical environment, policies and regulations, and transportation. An effective community physical activity intervention might also include such components as promotions, marketing, and complementary family programs. Using the ecological model allows program planners to simultaneously focus on multiple levels of influence around a child, increasing an intervention program's ability to address the various factors that appear to affect physical activity behavior. Table 5.1 illustrates how the ecological model can be applied to interventions that occur in the community.

Table 5.1 Ecological Approach to Organizing Theory Constructs in Community Settings

INFLUENCES ON BEHAVIOR	APPLICATION FOR INTERVENTIONS
Individual	
• Perceived self-efficacy • Expectations (including perceived benefits and barriers) • Intention to be physically active • Behavioral skills • Behavioral capability	• Instruction sessions (kick boxing, soccer clinics) held at settings like YMCA/YWCA • Dance performances held at the community center • Self-monitoring of pedometer steps to earn a Scout merit badge
Interpersonal	
• Social environment from social cognitive theory (including modeling and observational learning) • Social support/Social network • Social influence approaches	• Age- and/or gender-based sport teams or clubs • Mother-daughter or family-based activities • Exercise buddies at the community center
Organizational	
• Organizational change • Policies	• Physical activities included in community settings like churches as a regular part of family night services • Staff training sponsored by community recreation center on how to increase the number of sport programs for girls
Community	
• Interorganizational relations • Community development • Advocacy approaches	• Walking trail built around perimeter of Boys & Girls Club • Workshop with town council to improve walking connector between middle school and recreation center

Organizing Community Interventions

Community physical activity interventions can be organized around a single purpose, such as the promotion of physical activity in youth or decreased inactivity through encouraging youth to watch less television. Some community interventions are more complex and focus on such multiple outcomes as diet and physical activity behavior. Programs that attempt to intervene directly on a health outcome, such as decreasing or preventing overweight in children, are the most complex and intensive. To make a measurable impact, great effort, resources, and often multiple years of intervention may be required. This chapter includes these more comprehensive, and often more costly, interventions because the information might be useful for the development of new and less elaborate physical activity interventions.

Two approaches can be taken to design community physical activity interventions for children or adolescents. One approach is for interested organizations such as a university or government agency to organize, sponsor, and administer a program. Such an effort would be considered a physical activity program located in the community. The other approach is for interested organizations to partner and conduct the intervention collaboratively. This approach would be considered a physical activity program conducted with the community. Advantages of the first approach include expediency and control, whereas the second approach gets high marks for local identity and sustainability. Development of a program located in the community consists of finding an appropriate location, collecting local information, designing a community-specific program, and implementing the program for a specified period of time. Examples of such programs are provided in later sections of this chapter.

Ideally, community groups should be involved in designing programs and environments in order to provide the best opportunities for physical activity. Table 5.2 lists goals for community physical activity programs and guidelines for their achievement adapted from Guidelines for a Comprehensive Program to Promote Healthy Eating and Physical Activity (Nutrition and Physical Activity Work Group, 2002). The following sections describe successful community physical activity interventions that represent the types just outlined. The number of community interventions with young people is limited, so some of the programs described may not yet have been proven effective; but all have great promise.

Descriptions of Successful Community Interventions

The community offers a wide range of physical activity settings and opportunities for collaboration with many potential partners. The following are examples of successful community interventions organized by the type of community organization involved. These programs are summarized in

Table 5.2   Guidelines and Goals for Community Physical Activity Programs

GUIDELINES	GOALS
1. Increase number of community members and organizations involved in planning, conducting, and advocating for youth community programs.	1. Provide opportunities to learn how to be active.
2. Involve other members of the community who provide support for community programs, such as transportation, parks, and land use planning.	2. Provide safe environments for physical activity.
3. Organize groups who are often left out of consideration (low-income or minority groups).	3. Provide accessible and affordable opportunities for all youth to be active.
4. Promote adoption of physical activity policies and community infrastructure (sidewalks or school locations).	4. Eliminate disparities in support and resources for physical activity.

Adapted from Nutrition and Physical Activity Work Group, 2002.

the table "Summary of Basic Elements for Community-Based Programs" at the end of the chapter.

Day Care or Preschool Programs

The interventions described in this section are Nutrition and Physical Activity Self-Assessment for Child Care (NAP SACC) and Hip Hop to Health, Jr.

NAP SACC: Nutrition and Physical Activity Self-Assessment for Child Care

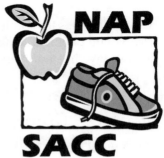

The NAP SACC program was an intervention that used professional facilitators such as health educators and child care consultants to help child care providers improve physical activity and nutrition at their centers (Story, Kaphingst, & French, 2006). Based on social cognitive theory, this program included a self-assessment tool for child care center directors and resources for the facilitator to use for technical assistance. The NAP SACC assessment instrument was used to assist in identifying strengths and challenges of healthy eating and physical activity in child care settings. A copy of the NAP SACC self-assessment instrument is located in appendix 5.A. In addition to the NAP SACC assessment instrument, the program provided a notebook with consultation guides and handouts for center staff and parents, as well as workshops on childhood overweight, healthy eating, physical activity, and staff wellness to be used to provide continuing education to child care staff. Consultants and child care center staff found a number of suggestions regarding why and how to improve in such areas as modeling physical activity and controlling television viewing, as well as resources with which to implement change. Each topic included information on how to get children to comply and how to involve parents in making changes at home. Preliminary results indicate that the NAP SACC intervention holds great promise for improving the physical activity and nutrition environments at child care centers. More information on this program can be found on the NAP SACC Web site (www.napsacc.org).

Hip Hop to Health, Jr.

Hip Hop to Health, Jr. was an obesity prevention program for preschool African American and Latino children based on Hip Hop to Health (see next section) and was tested in Head Start programs in Chicago (Fitzgibbon et al., 2002). The intervention was based on social cognitive theory, self-determination theory, and stages of change theory. The 14-week program was developmentally and culturally appropriate and took into account the language needs of attendees. The two components of this program were a weekly 20-minute lesson that covered either physical activity or healthy eating behaviors and two 20-minute sessions of physical activity. In addition to the classroom intervention, parents were sent weekly newsletters that provided the same information being taught to their children and that assigned homework for the parents to complete. Results of this intervention (Fitzgibbon et al., 2005) indicate that Hip Hop to Health, Jr. was successful in reducing the increases in body mass index often seen as children grow and develop. It was equally effective for girls and boys, and all children regardless of weight were positively affected.

Community Programs at School

Most physical activity interventions for youth have taken place within the school setting during school hours. Several of these interventions, however, have included an after-school component or have been adapted for use during the after-school period. Examples of the latter are described next.

SPARK After School

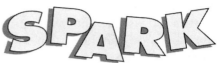

This program was developed as an offshoot of the Sports, Play and Active Recreation for Kids (SPARK) intervention, which is detailed in chapter 4 (Sallis et al., 1997). This variation on the SPARK program was developed for all out-of-school physical activity programs such as after-school, YMCA, Boys & Girls Clubs, recreation centers, day care centers, and camps. SPARK After School involves information and resources for project planners, training workshops for project staff, and follow-up support for participants and planners. Further details on the program and contact information are available on the SPARK Web site (www.sparkpe.org/programAfterSchool.jsp).

CKC: CATCH Kids Club

CATCH Kids Club was a physical activity and nutrition education program designed for elementary school children in grades K through 5, provided in an after-school or summer setting (Kelder et al., 2005). CKC, developed based on social cognitive theory, used elements of the Coordinated Approach to Child Health (CATCH) intervention, which is described in chapter 4. This program was designed to intervene on three elements: education, physical activity, and nutrition. The education component consisted of five modules targeted at K through second graders and third through fifth graders and was designed to increase children's self-efficacy, knowledge, and skills in nutritional and activity behaviors. One new lesson was provided each week for 15 to 30 minutes, and each lesson was designed to be fun and entertaining. The physical activity component included ideas for program leaders that were age appropriate, fun, and inclusive of all students in order to involve students in physical activity for at least 30 minutes each day, encourage students to participate in moderate-to-vigorous physical activity for at least 40% of that time, and provide students with a variety of enjoyable physical activity opportunities in order to build skills for the future. Lastly, healthy snacks were incorporated into the educational lessons in order to increase students' ability to prepare healthy snacks for themselves. Although the results of the educational portion of this intervention were equivocal, students were enthusiastic about their new snacks, and the physical activity component was a success. CKC increased children's moderate-to-vigorous physical activity from 30% to 57%, indicating that changes can be made to after-school programs to increase activity behaviors.

M-SPAN: Middle School Physical Activity and Nutrition

M-SPAN was an intervention designed to use environmental, policy, and social marketing approaches to increase physical activity and improve nutrition in middle school youth (Sallis et al., 2003). As noted in chapter 4, this was a comprehensive school intervention, but it also contained elements of a community program. Physical activity opportunities were offered before, during, and after school. Providers of physical activity (volunteers and some paid staff) came into the schools to offer programs, and additional activity equipment was provided. For an in-depth discussion of M-SPAN, see chapter 4.

TAAG: Trial of Activity for Adolescent Girls

TAAG, a multisite intervention designed to prevent the decline in physical activity in middle school girls, is another example of a comprehensive school-based intervention that includes a community component (Stevens et al., 2005). As of this book's publication, the TAAG intervention has not been 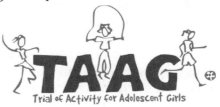 fully tested but includes useful ideas for increasing physical activity opportunities at school and in the community. For a fuller description of the TAAG intervention, see chapter 4 or the program's Web site (www. cscc.unc.edu/taag/).

Community Programs in Nonschool Settings

Several programs are described in this section, including Hip Hop to Health, Daughters and Mothers Exercising Together (DAMET), Go Girls, Girls Rule!, and Girl's health Enrichment Multi-site Studies (GEMS).

Hip Hop to Health

Hip Hop to Health was a culturally specific obesity prevention program designed for low-income, inner city African American girls (6-10 years old) and their mothers (Stolley & Fitzgibbon, 1997). This intervention stressed the importance of eating a low-fat, low-cholesterol diet and increasing physical activity. The idea for the intervention was taken from a highly successful community tutoring program. Mothers and daughters attended separate hourly sessions once per week at which they were exposed to a culturally specific obesity prevention program that encouraged them to eat low-fat, low-calorie diets and to increase their physical activity. In the physical activity component, culturally appropriate music and dance were used in a number of exercise- and diet-related educational experiences. For example, participants learned to sing and dance to raps against fat. Over the course of the 12-week program, only a few of the topics dealt with physical activity. However, results from the pilot program lend encouragement to the idea of including more intensive exercise components.

DAMET: Daughters and Mothers Exercising Together

DAMET was a mother-daughter (adolescent) physical activity intervention that included both classroom sessions and additional physical activity sessions attended by the mother-daughter pair twice per week (Ransdell et al., 2003). This program used social cognitive theory to develop 12 educational sessions. Although initial findings did not show changes in physical activity behavior, there were positive changes in physical self-perception and perceptions about physical activity (Ransdell, Detling, Taylor, Reel, & Shultz, 2004; Ransdell et al., 2005).

Go Girls

Go Girls was designed as a six-month intervention for African American adolescent girls living in public housing (Resnicow et al., 2000). Small groups of girls met once or twice weekly after school and participated in some field trips on weekends and holidays. Based on social cognitive theory, the sessions included knowledge and skill development. The varied physical activities included hip-hop/funk aerobics and "Afrobics," an aerobics program using hip-hop music or live drumming. A primary objective of the physical activity component was to expose girls to a wide variety of physical activity options. This project is still in an early stage of development, and no information is currently available regarding its effectiveness in changing physical activity behavior. However, the program design is promising because it uses culturally sensitive approaches to target the African American community and because the intervention is delivered where the girls live.

Girls Rule!

Girls Rule! was developed as a pilot program to intervene on physical activity and nutrition. The goal of Girls Rule! was to prevent overweight among 6- to 9-year-old girls by engaging the girls and their primary female caregivers. Girls met weekly at their churches for classes that included nutrition education and physical activities. Self-esteem activities were included as well. Primary caregivers (mothers or grandmothers) met twice per month: once as a group by themselves, and once with the girls. Each session included physical activity that was fun and had a practice/master/performance element (rope skipping, hula-hooping, or dancing) and emphasized practice at home. Sessions were designed to have an impact on personal factors, including self-efficacy, attitudes, and beliefs. Excursions or field trips were used to expose the girls to enjoyable ways to be physically active. Environmental support was available in the home and through the church; this included home visits, increased physical activity opportunities at the church, and addressing church policies to make them supportive of physical activity. This promising program should provide a rich opportunity to influence physical activity behavior in young girls. Girls Rule! finished its initial trial; and although no conclusive evidence is available, components of the program are of interest to those working with young girls or in church-based settings. Contact information for the Girls Rule! researchers can be found on the program's Web site (www.sph.unc.edu/nutr/about/girls_rule.htm).

GEMS: Girls Health Enrichment Multi-Site Studies

GEMS are pilot intervention studies based on social cognitive theory and are designed to prevent weight gain among young (prepubescent) African American girls. Four geographic sites developed GEMS programs, all with different approaches to healthy eating and physical activity. An entire issue of the journal *Ethnicity and Disease* (Vol. 13, Suppl. 1, 2003) was dedicated to the GEMS project and detailed the physical activity components of the four studies led by universities across the country (Baylor, Memphis, Minnesota, and Stanford).

Baylor GEMS used a summer camp format and a number of approaches to increase physical activity (Baranowski et al., 2003). Girls were taught dance skills, and pedometers were used for self-monitoring. The means of engaging parents was to teach the girls to ask their parents to be active with them, and a buddy system to encourage physical activity was used.

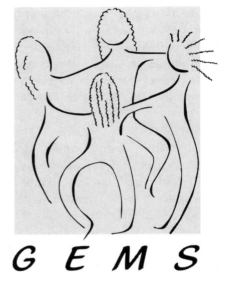

G E M S

Girls health Enrichment Multi-Site Program

Memphis GEMS used two intervention approaches: girl-only and parent-only. The girl-only approach included activities that the girls suggested were fun. Hip-hop aerobics and dancing during television commercials were two activities used. In the parent-only approach, parents and caregivers danced to popular songs from the 70s and 80s in 25-minute dance segments. The two groups were encouraged to share their dance interests with each other (Beech et al., 2003).

Minnesota GEMS used a club meeting format in which "members" met for 1 hour twice per week after school. Meetings included a choice from a variety of physical activities, such as dancing, double-dutch jump rope, and other culturally appropriate games. Families received take home packets of information, participated in activities such as family night events, and received encouragement telephone calls (Story et al., 2003).

Stanford GEMS used an after-school dance class format and included a component for reducing TV watching. The dance classes were held five days per week at community centers over the 12-week period. An educational program on TV reduction was delivered through home visits, and an electronic TV time manager was used to create time allowances for television viewing (Robinson et al., 2003).

At the time of this book's publication, only preliminary findings about these four GEMS programs were available. However, the GEMS studies represent innovative interventions that could be adapted for use by others.

In chapter 7, the basic elements for physical activity program planning are discussed, including the target group for the program, cooperating professionals (change agents), the type of physical activity behavior to be changed, and where and when the program will take place. Table 5.3 at the end of the chapter shows these basic elements, as well as program components, for the interventions just described.

Working in and With Communities

It is sometimes difficult to work with a local community to identify a need or opportunity, plan collaboratively, and implement a community physical activity program. Working alone or with individuals who think similarly and have similar beliefs and skills is much easier than accommodating the varied backgrounds, needs, interests, and skills of local community members. The long-term benefits of collaboration or partnership, however, may be great. Unfortunately, few partnership programs have been developed, and fewer still have found their way into the public domain (Minkler & Wallerstein, 2002). Table 5.3 presents a list of the key issues for understanding interventions in community settings. Later in this book (chapter 7), we present information on planning and involving community stakeholders.

You must consider several challenges when designing physical activity interventions for youth in community settings, including understanding the community and identifying appropriate partners, defining the scope of the program and the purpose of collaboration, forming effective working relationships with community partners, and creating a positive focus. The following are tips for working in collaboration with community groups or agencies.

Learn the Community Context

It is not a good idea to rush into a community setting with your programs and solutions to their problems. Identify first what the community sees as a problem and what solutions are currently available. Find out what is going on, what is working, and what has not worked, and express your collaborative intention to build on strengths. To avoid unintentionally insulting community individuals and groups, get to know the community, the local agencies, and the organizations, and invite potential players to

Table 5.3 Key Issues in Understanding Interventions in Community Settings

ISSUE	EXPLANATION
1. Target audiences involved	
	• Single primary target (e.g., adolescents) with other groups (e.g., parents) involved to help with the primary target
	• Multiple targets (e.g., children, adolescents, and parents) with an equal focus on each
	Interventions in community settings traditionally involve multiple target groups.
2. Origin of community program	
	Idea for program arises from within the community and:
	• Community members take charge of the program
	• Experts may be sought for assistance
	Idea for program arises from outside the community and:
	• Outside "expert group" takes charge of the program
	• Outside group must work toward obtaining community "buy-in" for the issue
3. Involvement of community members in planning, implementing, and evaluating program	
	Two extremes:
	• Outsiders bring a program already largely developed and attempt to implement and evaluate it without community participation.
	• Program is developed, carried out, and evaluated collaboratively with community members.
	Many programs fall between these two extremes.
4. Focus on community needs versus community strengths	
	Needs focus:
	• Identifies health problem (e.g., obesity) or risk behavior (e.g., physical inactivity)
	• Develops strategy to reduce or minimize the problem in the target group
	Strengths focus:
	• Identifies what is working
	• Further develops capacities and skills
	A program can employ elements of both of these approaches
5. Primary types of strategies used	
	• Consensus and collaboration (community organization and development)
	• Confrontation and conflict (social action) to foster change
	The latter is used when power is unequally distributed.

become involved. Be prepared to devote some time to planning; the extra effort will be highly worthwhile.

Define Program Scope and Purpose With Community Partners

Identify the target audience(s), change agent(s), and target behavior(s) for the program, but be realistic. Remember that including multiple audiences, multiple behaviors, and a variety of strategies might require more money and time. Talk early and openly about how the partner agencies, organizations, and groups will work together. Common questions that should be asked include the following:

- Are the intervention planners interested in working with an organization primarily to gain entry to a group of kids? For example, a community center or church recreation group might serve as a platform through which physical activity programs can be offered.
- Are the planners primarily interested in getting input, ideas, and cooperation so that potential participants and referral sources will support the program?
- Are the planners interested in a partnership that involves collaboration to develop and carry out the program?

Expectations should be clearly defined. Different partners (agencies, groups, and organizations) will play different roles, such as contribution of tangible resources, including funds, equipment, and space; coordination and communication; program promotion and participant recruitment; provision or facilitation of transportation; and adult supervision and program delivery.

Establish Effective Partner Relationships

Get to know all partners and ask questions. What is a typical work day like in the partner organization? What are the priorities and policies that might affect collaboration with that organization? Establish an identity as a group and work toward developing cohesion. Seek agreement from partners on these common goals and develop an effective working structure among all partners, including working committees, communications, ongoing leadership, decision-making procedures, and establishment of meaningful roles for all partners. Work through conflicts openly and use them as a means to develop the group. Expect and accept changes in partner members and the roles they play if the program continues over an extended period of time.

Aim for a Positive Focus

Work on potentially demoralizing problem areas such as health problems and lack of resources, and be prepared if these situations arise. Consider the strengths as well as the weaknesses of the community. Ask how the talents of youth, parents, older adults, and others in the community can be used in a positive way or how the accomplishments and potential of agencies, groups, and organizations can help the program. If barriers seem insurmountable, focus on what "could be." Redefine barriers as challenges and avoid becoming preoccupied with day-to-day details.

SUMMARY

Communities can provide rich and varied opportunities for youth physical activity. When planning community interventions, it is most effective to consider whether the program will be planned in the community or planned with the community. It might seem easier to plan programs independently; but for implementation and sustainability, working with the community might be best. Community physical activity programs can be implemented in a wide range of settings such as churches, community centers, preschools, and housing developments. Engaging adults to work with youth has been found to be useful as well. Regardless of site, communities are great places to promote, encourage, and reinforce physical activity in young people.

Summary of Basic Elements for Community-Based Programs

INTERVENTION	TARGET	CHANGE AGENTS	PROGRAM COMPONENTS	PHYSICAL ACTIVITY (PA) BEHAVIOR
Day care/Preschool				
NAP SACC	Preschool children, ages 2-5 years	Preschool provider	Self-assessment instrument; action plan for improvement; technical assistance to change environment.	General PA
Hip Hop for Health, Jr.	Preschool children in Head Start	Preschool provider	Classes for children on nutrition and PA; parent component.	General PA
School				
SPARK After School	Middle school youth	After-school professionals	Activities that include SPARK physical education components can be used in after-school programs.	Fitness and MVPA
M-SPAN	Middle school youth	After-school professionals	Community component has providers who bring programs to school.	MVPA
CATCH Kids Club	Elementary school children	After-school professionals	Uses CATCH principles to develop improved after-school programs.	MVPA

(continued)

Summary of Basic Elements for Community-Based Programs *(continued)*

INTERVENTION	TARGET	CHANGE AGENTS	PROGRAM COMPONENTS	PHYSICAL ACTIVITY (PA) BEHAVIOR
Nonschool				
Hip Hop for Health	6- to 10-year-old girls	Research staff and mothers	Program includes use of culturally appropriate physical activities.	General PA, MVPA
Go Girls	Adolescent girls	Research staff	Program includes use of culturally appropriate physical activities.	General PA
Girls Rule!	Young girls	Mothers and church staff	Age-appropriate physical activities at church for girls and aerobics for moms.	MVPA
DAMET	Adolescent girls	Mothers	12-week program that included weekly exercise activities performed together.	Health-related physical fitness
GEMS	Preadolescent African American girls	Mothers, research staff, or both	Culturally appropriate activities from dance to jump rope and games.	MVPA

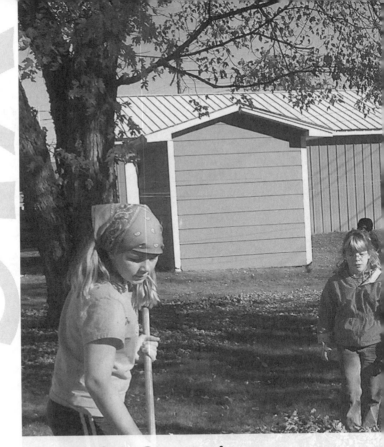

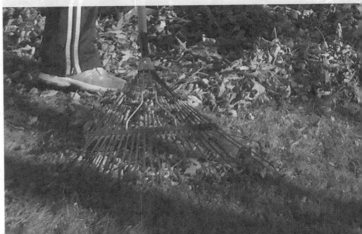

SIX

Family-Based Interventions in Home and Health Care Settings

Evidence from previous research studies has shown that families provide key support for youth activity. In this chapter, we present information on specific interventions that have focused on families, as well as program ideas that can be used to optimize the role of family members in the adoption of physical activity behaviors in children and adolescents. In addition, we describe specific behaviors of parents and family members that have been shown to influence physical activity in youth.

Making the Most of Home and Health Care Settings

For the purpose of this chapter, the home is a private setting in which physical activity can be facilitated by parents, guardians, or caretakers. A health care setting might be a doctor's office, and physical activity in this type of setting would be facilitated by both clinicians and family members. Physical activity programs that target these two types of settings are often called family-based interventions because the parents or primary caretakers are involved in children's physical activity. This term is used for the rest of the chapter to refer to interventions that focus on children in home and health care settings. School interventions also sometimes have family components, but these intervention approaches were covered in chapter 4.

CDC Recommendation 6

Parental involvement: Include parents and guardians in physical activity instruction and in extracurricular and community physical activity programs, and encourage them to support their children's participation in enjoyable physical activities.

(CDC, 1997)

The role of families and health providers was highlighted in the Centers for Disease Control and Prevention publication, "Guidelines for School and Community Programs to Support Physical Activity Among Young People" (CDC, 1997). The CDC's guideline for parental involvement appears in the sidebar. Involvement in physical activity programs provides opportunities for parents to be partners in developing their children's physical activity-related knowledge, attitudes, motor skills, behavioral skills, confidence, and behavior. Family involvement can be encouraged by teachers, coaches, and other school officials, as well as health care professionals. In school-based interventions, teachers can assign homework or provide flyers designed for parents that contain information and strategies for promoting physical activity within the family.

In addition to the direct role of parents in developing physical activity behaviors in their children, some parents decide to consult or engage physicians, psychologists, nutritionists, and other health care professionals in addressing the particular health needs of their child. These professionals have an opportunity to affect physical activity through direct youth–provider interaction or by discussing with parents how best to support children's activity. The CDC's recommendation for involvement of health service professionals is shown in the sidebar. Health care providers are important in promoting physical activity, especially among children and adolescents who have physical or cognitive disabilities or chronic health conditions. Young people and their families should be counseled about the importance of physical activity and should be given information that enables them to initiate and maintain regular, safe, and enjoyable participation in physical activity (CDC, 1997).

CDC Recommendation 8

Health services: Assess physical activity patterns among young people, counsel them about physical activity, refer them to appropriate programs, and advocate for physical activity instruction and programs for young people.
(CDC, 1997)

Organizing Family-Based Interventions

Family-based interventions can be implemented as part of routine family activities, through changes in the household environment, or through professional guidance from health care providers. Parents and guardians, as well as siblings and relatives, may initiate physical activity programs at home. In addition, parents' roles as facilitators of physical activity in children can be capitalized on through routine medical or specialized health care treatment programs that help parents learn to help their children. Physicians, school nurses, nurse practitioners, or psychologists can provide targeted interventions to families in their care, and these family members then become agents of change at home. Although few family-based and health care-based programs currently exist, the need for effective at-home interventions to address special health needs (e.g., of children with asthma or those who are overweight) will require a greater focus on such initiatives in the design of future interventions.

Family involvement is often used in large, multicomponent interventions along with other intervention components. For example, a school-based program like CATCH included a parent component that used take-home newsletters or homework assistance to focus on raising parent awareness of physical activity participation. This chapter does not address interventions such as these since school interventions and community programs that include parent components were covered in chapters 4 and 5.

Other interventions in which parents serve as agents of change to promote children's physical activity include programs in the health care setting. Medical professionals might operate as a single provider (pediatrician, nutritionist, or psychologist) or as a member of a multidisciplinary team to address child or family physical activity behaviors, including those related to chronic health conditions like obesity or type 2 diabetes. These health care professionals can alert the youth or family members to a potential problem with the child's physical activity, provide counseling as to how to make necessary changes, and expect family members to implement family support and make appropriate changes in the home environment in support of physical activity.

Using Behavior Theory in Family-Based Interventions

Family-based interventions focus on the unique relationships between the young people and adults in a family. The family unit in which children live, the relationships between the youth and the adults, and their interactions regarding health and well-being are strong forces that constitute one of the most important influences on short- and long-term health behavior. Addressing the family is a fundamental approach to behavior change, but among the most difficult to organize and conduct. Hence, few family-based physical activity interventions exist.

Parents and family members have an enormous opportunity to influence a child's physical activity. Although the proportion is not specifically known, early parental influences clearly affect physical activity development and are separate from the genetic component that cannot be changed. As noted in previous chapters, many interventions include influences that affect physical activity on multiple levels, using an approach known as the ecological framework. A multilevel approach affords greater opportunity to influence behavior than an approach that depends on a single intervention strategy. Influences on children's physical activity behavior that are affected or facilitated by families can be organized using an ecological model as indicated in table 6.1.

Table 6.1 Ecological Approach to Organizing Theory Constructs in Family-Based Settings

INFLUENCES ON BEHAVIOR	APPLICATION FOR INTERVENTIONS
Individual	
• Perceived self-efficacy • Expectations (including perceived benefits and barriers) • Intention to be physically active • Behavioral skills • Behavioral capability	• Individual youth counseling sessions conducted by family doctor, nutritionist, or psychologist • Parent education skill-building sessions conducted by lay health advisor or health educator
Interpersonal	
• Social environment from social cognitive theory (including modeling and observational learning) • Social support/Social network • Social influence approaches	• Use of family member (parent, sibling) to support and/or facilitate physical activity • Families making house rules: TV time limited to 1 hour per day, or 30 minutes of physical activity daily required to watch 1 hour of TV • Group counseling sessions at the clinical site that include youth who share a common characteristic (such as overweight) • Mother-daughter or family-based activities for use at home
Organizational*	
• Organizational change • Policies	• Linking child-parent physical activity through school assignments • Family-friendly polices for use of school facilities (e.g., open gym in evening) • Work site health promotion program that includes family members, especially children

(continued)

Table 6.1 *(continued)*

INFLUENCES ON BEHAVIOR	APPLICATION FOR INTERVENTIONS
Community*	
• Interorganizational relations • Community development • Advocacy approaches	• Family-friendly walking trail built around perimeter of Boys & Girls Club • Community event that focuses on family physical activities, with physical activity promoted for all family members • Clinicians advocating for family physical activity opportunities at schools, at recreational centers, or in community groups

*Usually implemented through other settings such as school or community.

Many of the constructs applicable to family-based interventions fall within the interpersonal level of the ecological approach. Parents serve mainly as social support in providing encouragement, transportation, and involvement in physical activity (Gustafson & Rhodes, 2006). Verbal or nonverbal efforts, such as encouragement to play outside or to watch less TV, can help children to be active. Being encouraged by parents provides kids with the reassurance that they are able or competent to be active. Parents also provide help by engaging in activities with the child and practicing skills or playing games. Additionally, parents support their children's physical activity behaviors by doing such things as providing transportation or enrolling kids in sport programs. Finally, parents and other family members who themselves have regular physical activity behaviors influence a child's physical activity by being good role models for kids (Welk, 1999a). Although most parents who are active also encourage and support child activity, parents' physical activity level may not be as strongly related to child physical activity as is their support and facilitation (Gustafson & Rhodes, 2006).

Evaluating Home and Health Care Interventions

Behavior change is the purpose of all interventions, even those in family-based settings. Behavior theories, as described earlier, typically are used to ensure a more probable outcome. As noted previously, though, few examples of family-based interventions for physical activity are available.

Examples of programs that do exist are presented next, organized into home-based and health care-based interventions. Most of these targeted overweight youth, although the ideas could be used with children of any health status.

Home-Based Interventions

The home-based interventions we discuss here are DAMET—Daughters and Mothers Exercising Together; a family-monitored home exercise program; and two studies that sought to reduce TV viewing time.

DAMET: Daughters and Mothers Exercising Together

DAMET tested a mother-daughter exercise program implemented at two sites: a community fitness center and individual family homes (Ransdell et al., 2003). The two interventions were similar in structure. Information on the DAMET intervention is also presented in chapter 5. The unique contribution of this program to family interventions is the inclusion of a home-based exercise program. The home-based group received a detailed packet of information containing a calendar of recommended activities, pictures of particular exercises, and tips for overcoming barriers. Activities focused primarily on increasing aerobic fitness, muscle strength, and flexibility. Participants were faithful to the recommended procedures, and only three pairs (18% of study participants) dropped out. Results indicated that both the community- and the home-based programs were effective in changing many aspects of physical fitness, especially in the mothers. Girls significantly improved their muscular endurance. Programs of this type have great promise as an inexpensive intervention strategy.

Family-Monitored Home Exercise Program

Taggart and colleagues (1986) administered a fitness performance test to all children from one school who were enrolled in grades 4, 5, and 6. They identified 17 children as low-fit, and 12 of these children and their parents agreed to participate in the study. Children who were found to have low health fitness scores were prescribed a remedial exercise program by their physical education teacher. Parents, with support from the teacher, recorded baseline leisure-time physical activity levels during nonschool hours to ensure that children were performing activity for 10 minutes or longer and that the activity involved the whole body in movement.

The home-based behavioral program used a parent-determined reward system based on activity points accumulated, and the incentive changed over the intervention period to reward increasing physical activity. After implementation of this program, all of the enrolled children increased their physical activity from their baseline level; the increases ranged from 50% to 500%. An increase of nearly 50% was also found in number of minutes per week spent in activity. This program demonstrated that children, under the supervision of parents who could set appropriate goals and rewards for their child, could improve their health fitness levels.

Reducing TV Time

A number of interventions that center on reducing sedentary behaviors have been effective in decreasing inactivity and, in some cases, increasing physical activity. Success has been observed when TV viewing is targeted for reduction. Techniques for decreasing the amount of television viewing time have included both educational and environmental approaches. Educational approaches are successful when, for example, information is presented about television viewing, the school curriculum focuses on reducing time spent in front of the television, and substitute activities are offered. Environmental change approaches are successful when, for example, TV is limited by either family policies or by a mechanical device called a TV allowance box that monitors and prevents excessive TV watching.

Two studies of TV reduction offer examples of how sedentary behavior can be targeted. The first study was initiated at school but had a home component—use of the TV allowance box (Robinson, 1999). Third- and fourth-grade students in two California public elementary schools were recruited for this study. Students in the intervention group received in-class instruction on self-reporting television use, were challenged to watch no TV and play no video games for 10 days, and were encouraged to budget their TV time thereafter by being more selective about the programs they watched. Parents of students in the intervention group were given a TV allowance box to use at home to budget TV time. At the end of the program, students in the intervention group had statistically significant decreases in BMI, waist circumference, and triceps skinfold thickness, as well as decreases in television viewing and video game use (Robinson, 1999).

The other study took place primarily at the physician's office but also included home use of a TV allowance box (Ford, McDonald, Owens, & Robinson, 2002). Clinic staff helped parents set up "budgets" for TV, videos, and computer game use. In families that received standard counseling about ways to increase physical activity and received a TV allowance box, children's media use (TV, videos, and video games) decreased by nearly 14 hours per week, while physical activity time (playing outside and engaging in organized activity) increased by close to 3 hours per week. Those families who did not receive the intervention showed a reduction in the number of hours of physical activity time for children. The results from this study indicate that although limiting TV time might contribute to an increase in physical activity time for children, television viewing is not the only barrier to physical activity.

Health Care-Based Interventions

The health care-based interventions we discuss here are a pedometer goal program for earning the reward of sedentary pursuits and the PACE+ program for increasing moderate-to-vigorous physical activity.

Contingency Management to Increase Activity and Decrease Inactivity

An understanding of how children make decisions can be used to increase physical activity. This approach, called behavioral economics or contingency management, has been used to promote physical activity by decreasing sedentary pursuits or by linking activity to a reinforcement or reward (Epstein, 1998). Many sedentary activities such as watching television or videos or playing computer games are easier to accomplish than finding a friend to play with or riding a bike when it is hot outside. In work with low-fit or overweight youth, successful interventions have been conducted that target sedentary behaviors. These studies have shown that when children are reinforced for reducing sedentary behavior, not only does inactivity time decrease, but children correspondingly increase their activity time. Sedentary pursuits are easy to find, and many youth, especially those who are overweight, have clear preferences for inactive options. Because activity is not their first choice, programs that promote physical activities might not be immediately embraced by these youth. However, when children are reinforced for avoiding inactive pursuits, it is their choice as to what types of activities they engage in instead. Thus, behavioral economics, based on behavioral choice theory (Epstein, 1998), allows children to decide how to "spend" their time. Reinforcing less time spent in sedentary activities provides a stimulus for the substitute—a physically active option—to be chosen by the child herself (Epstein,

Roemmich, Paluch, & Raynor, 2005).

Two types of approaches have been used in behavioral economics: closed loop and open loop feedback. Closed loop feedback means that the target behavior is tied directly to the preferred activity. For example, a closed loop approach links a health behavior desired by adults (physical activity) to an activity desired by children (watching TV). One example of this approach consisted of a stationary bike connected to a TV. The TV required "foot-powered electricity" for the viewing of programs (Faith et al., 2001). When the TV could be watched only during cycling, the amount of pedaling time was 64.4 minutes per week, and the amount of TV watched was 1.6 hours per week. This compared to 8.3 minutes of pedaling and 21.0 hours of TV per week when the bike and TV were both available but not hooked together. The closed loop approach shows good promise in encouraging children to select health-promoting options.

A more flexible method that targets behavioral choices is called open loop feedback. In this approach, another person such as a parent determines if the activity goals have been reached and whether the reinforcement or reward should be provided. In an example of open loop feedback, overweight children were assigned to groups based on different goals for accumulating pedometer steps: 1500 steps, 750 steps, and zero steps (control group) (Goldfield, Kalakanis, Ernst, & Epstein, 2000). Placed in a room with different exercise equipment and many sedentary options (TV, video, books, computer games), children could earn time for sedentary options if they achieved the pedometer goals that had been set. Children in the control group could freely use either the active or the sedentary choices. The children in the highest step group performed more physical activity than did the children in the lower goal or control group. Although this study was conducted in a more research-like setting, the approach indicates that physical activity can be used to earn access to desirable sedentary pursuits.

PACE+

Few physician-based programs have been developed specifically to increase youth physical activity. One program that shows great promise is PACE+ (Patrick et al., 2001; Prochaska, Zabinski, Calfas, Sallis, & Patrick, 2000). PACE+ was based on a successful adult-focused

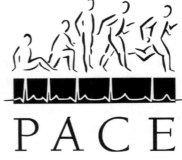

clinical counseling program called PACE, Patient-Centered Counseling for Exercise. PACE+ focused on four health behaviors: (1) total dietary fat consumption, (2) fruit and vegetable consumption, (3) moderate and vigorous physical activity, and (4) sedentary activity. Using the stages of change theory, the program involved computerized behavior assessment and goal setting, counseling by a health care provider, and extensive manual-based telephone counseling and mail outreach regarding the youth's readiness to undertake change. Phone counseling along with print materials guided adolescents to use cognitive and behavioral skills to make changes in behaviors. PACE+ also used time in the waiting room to employ a computer-based assessment and counseling model that identified motivators for behavior change and developed a self-change plan incorporating goal-setting, social support, and problem-solving techniques to change or maintain one physical activity and one nutrition behavior.

In both boys and girls, sedentary time decreased by about 1 hour per day (Patrick et al., 2006). The number of boys meeting the physical activity recommendation (30 minutes of vigorous or 60 minutes of moderate-to-vigorous physical activity) increased as well. Adolescents appeared highly satisfied with all components of the program, providing evidence that the program is a feasible way to offer interactive physical activity and nutritional health communication to adolescents in a primary care setting. Further information on PACE and PACE+ can be found on the program's Web site (www.paceproject.org).

The summary table at the end of the chapter lists the interventions described in this chapter and identifies the basic elements and program components contained in these home-based and health care-based interventions for youth.

Working With Families in Home and Health Care Settings

If you wish to target your intervention at a home or health care setting, it is necessary first to develop effective collaboration with parents or caregivers. Parents are in a unique position to influence the health of their children. Parents set the stage for health behaviors, provide reinforcement for such behavior, and serve as emotional supports in the behavior change process. In an intervention, parents can serve three roles: providing support, serving as role models, and setting limits.

Providing Support

Most children like to be active, but often something more is needed to make it happen. Parents can provide tangible assistance, sometimes called instrumental support, for children to engage in physical activities. In order to find a safe place to ride a bike, it might be necessary to drive the child to a park or field. Enrolling youth in sport programs or paying for tennis lessons can also aid in the child's quest for an active life. Family support is important for sustaining a child's interest in activity. Attending games, watching pickup play in the backyard, asking questions, and generally demonstrating interest add support to the youth's participation in physical activity (Gustafson & Rhodes, 2006).

Role Modeling

Active adults present a consistent and enduring reminder of the role of physical activity in health and happiness. Parents and guardians who participate in exercise or activity have children who are more likely to be active (Trost, Kerr, Ward, & Pate, 2001; Sallis et al., 1992). It is not important, however, to be athletic, to engage in any specialized sports, or to be a highly successful performer (Sallis, Prochaska, & Taylor, 2000). Regular walking (with the dog or with others), working in the yard, and doing living room calisthenics illustrate the role physical activity plays in the life of an adult. With the knowledge that role modeling might influence child behavior, negative behavior must be considered as well (Fogelholm, Nuutinen, Pasanen, Myöhänen, & Säätelä, 1999). Fathers who spend much of their time after work in front of the TV and mothers who do not have a regular physical activity pattern might present an adverse model for their offspring. Care should be taken to minimize negative role modeling. Parental involvement has been shown to be particularly relevant for girls, as evidenced by the impact of parental activity levels and parental encouragement. It has been shown that mothers provide greater support and facilitation for physical activity, while fathers tend to demonstrate personal involvement in the activity (Davison, Cutting, & Birch, 2003).

Although it seems logical that children who see active parents would be inclined to imitate them, demonstrated support for physical activity is more important. Work by Welk and colleagues (Welk, Wood, & Morss, 2003; Welk, 1999b) showed that parental facilitation, encouragement, and involvement were more important to a child's physical activity participation than role modeling an active lifestyle. Role modeling was useful, but primarily as a function of support. More active parents tended to provide more support for the physical activities of their children (Gustafson & Rhodes, 2006).

Setting Limits

Parents play important roles in a child's activity level not only through promoting physical activity, but also through their efforts to minimize inactivity. Requiring a child to be active might, in the long run, be an ineffective way to create positive feelings about physical activity. It is often easier to set household rules or policies focusing on household objects that create inactivity than to try to force kids to be active. One example is to limit the amount of TV viewing allowed through a TV viewing policy. The average American child spends nearly 6 hours per day watching television and using other electronic media such as video games and computers (Roberts, Foehr, Rideout, & Brodie, 1999)! The relationship between inactivity and physical activity seems to be one of opposite behaviors. Decreasing the time spent in sedentary pursuits such as watching TV, playing computer games, or watching videos will surely provide more time for active pursuits. However, the choice between physical activity and sedentary pursuits seems to respond to different stimuli (Ford et al., 2002). Screen time plays a major role in the sedentary behavior of American youth. Parents and guardians can monitor and control children's and adolescents' access to the TV and computer; and, as already discussed, family-based programs to support such behaviors exist.

Defining Roles for Health Care Professionals

Health care professionals can also play numerous roles in physical activity interventions. They can assume the role of primary change agents, working directly with the youth; they can be change agents in their work to educate or "coach" parents who would then be secondary targets of an intervention; or they can assume the role of advocate.

• **Counseling youth.** Depending on the age of the child, health care professionals can directly interact with youth to counsel them regarding an active lifestyle. Although the impact of clinicians on physical activity behavior in youth has not been well studied, such interaction might be a useful approach with older youth or with youth who have a chronic disease.

- **Coaching parents.** Health care providers, especially physicians, can play a significant role in motivating parents to support healthy child behavior. It may be, however, that this influence is not exerted because of the physician's discomfort in initiating discussions with parents on health issues that require increased physical activity in their children, such as weight problems. Few resources are currently available to the physician on how to counsel or coach parents to serve as health educators for their children. Helping parents help their children engage in regular physical activity might require working to get the entire family physically active.

- **Becoming advocates.** Clinicians and other health care professionals can play a key role in promoting physical activity for youth. These community leaders can advocate for school and community physical activity instruction and programs that meet the needs of young people. To help create physical and social environments that encourage physical activity, health care providers should advocate for physical education curricula, extracurricular activities, and community sport and recreation programs that emphasize lifetime physical activities and that enable participation in safe, enjoyable physical activities.

Physicians, school nurses, and other health care professionals can support physical activity among children and adolescents by becoming involved in school and community physical activity initiatives. Physicians can volunteer to serve as advisors to schools and other community organizations that provide physical activity programs and facilities for young people. Health care providers should advocate that coaches be trained to ensure that young people compete safely and thrive physically, emotionally, and socially. Chapter 5 includes specific information on community-based interventions involving the physician as advocate.

The different roles that parents and health care providers can play in encouraging physical activity in youth are summarized in table 6.2.

Table 6.2 Parent and Health Care Provider Roles in Physical Activity

ROLE OF PARENTS	ROLE OF HEALTH CARE PROVIDERS
1. Providing emotional and tangible support for children to engage in physical activities 2. Role modeling physical activity behaviors themselves 3. Setting limits to sedentary activities in which their children engage	1. Counseling youth on physical activity behaviors 2. Coaching parents to motivate their child's active pursuits 3. Becoming advocates in schools and communities for physical activity programs

SUMMARY

Families exert a strong influence over children's and adolescents' lives. Although few home-based interventions for physical activity exist, a number of useful ideas have been employed either as part of larger interventions or as stand-alone programs. Sometimes youth need assistance from health care personnel to address problems such as obesity. Programs based in physicians' offices that are supervised at home by parents have shown promise. Whether reduction of TV viewing or increased physical activity behavior is the focus, family-sponsored and family-supported interventions can help improve the lives of youth.

Summary of Basic Elements for Family-Based Interventions

INTERVENTION	TARGET	CHANGE AGENTS	PROGRAM COMPONENTS	PHYSICAL ACTIVITY BEHAVIOR
Home setting				
DAMET	14- to 17-year-old girls	Mothers	12-week home-based prescribed exercise program	Health fitness
Home fitness program	12-year-olds	Parents	9- to 22-week home-based prescribed exercise program	Health fitness

(continued)

Summary of Basic Elements for Family-Based Interventions *(continued)*

INTERVENTION	TARGET	CHANGE AGENTS	PROGRAM COMPONENTS	PHYSICAL ACTIVITY BEHAVIOR
Home setting *(continued)*				
Reducing TV time 1	8- to 9-year-olds	Teachers Parents	Eighteen 30- to 50-min lessons; TV turn-off; TV allowance box	TV viewing time MVPA
Reducing TV time 2	7- to 12-year-olds	Parents	5- to 10–min counseling; 15-20 min TV budgets; TV allowance box	TV viewing time MVPA
Cycling to watch TV	Obese 8- to 12-year-olds	Parents	12-week in-home study using specially designed TV cycle	MVPA
Health care setting				
Pedometer goals to earn sedentary activity time	8- to 12-year-olds	Contin-gency goal	Required to meet steps goal in order to "cash in" for sedentary play	MVPA
PACE+	11- to 15-year-olds	Clinician; computer-based material	Information on physical activity and sedentary behavior (along with nutrition information); goal setting	MVPA Sedentary time

Intervention
Design

three

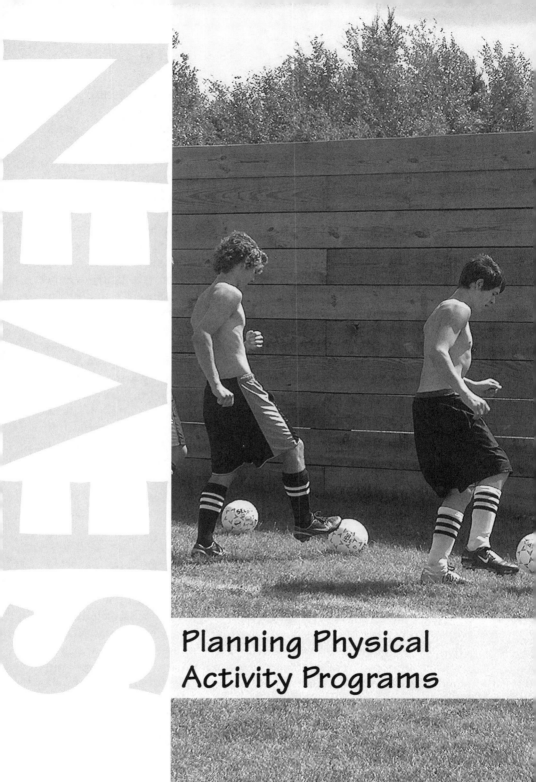

SEVEN

Planning Physical Activity Programs

In part I of this book, we introduced the nature of physical activity, theories about behavior, and settings in which to focus interventions. As noted in chapter 2, before planning an intervention, it is imperative to consider the population to be served, the site of the program, the type of physical activity, and the objectives of the program. Detailed information is presented in chapter 2 with respect to identifying behavior to be changed, listing influences on physical activity, selecting appropriate methods, and developing operational intervention strategies. A variety of effective interventions are presented in part II (chapters 4-6) as a consolidation of information about different physical activity settings and the methods and theoretical constructs applicable to their design.

The current chapter represents the beginning of part III, in which we describe steps for intervention planning, implementation, and evaluation. Helpful worksheets are provided in the appendix to aid in program design and organization. There are two phases for program design: the planning phase and the implementation phase. The planning phase includes both program planning (this chapter) and program evaluation planning (chapters 9 and 10). Even though they are discussed in separate chapters, it is important to understand that program planning and program evaluation planning are linked and are part of the same process. The implementation phase includes carrying out, monitoring, and evaluating the program (chapter 10). The planning and implementing phases can be broken down into six different steps, as shown in figure 7.1. The remainder of this chapter covers steps 1 and 2—how to identify support for a program and how to plan a program based on the needs of a population. Step 3 is covered in chapter 9, and steps 4 through 6 are covered in chapter 10.

Step 1: Identify and Engage Partners

Planning should begin with identifying and engaging the people who will be involved in putting on or supporting the program, as well as those who are served or affected by the program. These people might include financial supporters, sponsors, program planners, decision makers, program staff, program implementers, program participants, and other stakeholders. Identify those directly affected by the program who can provide useful input into the planning from their perspective. Teachers, for example, should be involved in planning programs implemented in school settings because their daily relationship with the target popula-

Planning phase

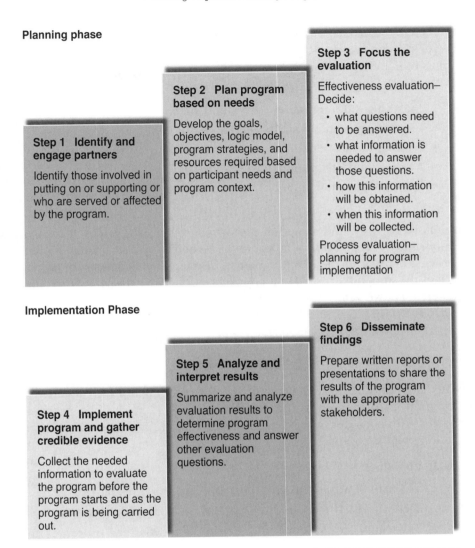

Step 1 Identify and engage partners

Identify those involved in putting on or supporting or who are served or affected by the program.

Step 2 Plan program based on needs

Develop the goals, objectives, logic model, program strategies, and resources required based on participant needs and program context.

Step 3 Focus the evaluation

Effectiveness evaluation–Decide:

• what questions need to be answered.
• what information is needed to answer those questions.
• how this information will be obtained.
• when this information will be collected.

Process evaluation–planning for program implementation

Implementation Phase

Step 4 Implement program and gather credible evidence

Collect the needed information to evaluate the program before the program starts and as the program is being carried out.

Step 5 Analyze and interpret results

Summarize and analyze evaluation results to determine program effectiveness and answer other evaluation questions.

Step 6 Disseminate findings

Prepare written reports or presentations to share the results of the program with the appropriate stakeholders.

Figure 7.1 Planning and implementing physical activity programs.

Adapted from the Centers for Disease Control and Prevention (CDC), 1999, and U.S. Department of Health and Human Services, 2002.

tion can provide insight into methods and theories that can be used in planning a program. In addition, input from those who will receive the program, such as the children themselves, should be considered. From this initial list, a group of planning partners can be formed.

It might seem easier and faster to create a program alone rather than to seek out and work with stakeholders; however, there are many advantages to planning and implementing physical activity programs through team effort. Some of these advantages are the following:

- Including different perspectives and skills
- Expanding contacts and potential resources
- Sharing the workload
- Increasing participation in the program
- Enhancing sustainability of the program

Building an effective team requires efforts from leaders who are comfortable with and skilled at performing tasks as a group. It is also important to keep group members involved and informed throughout the process of program planning, implementation, and evaluation. Worksheet 7.1 in the appendix provides a checklist of considerations for building an effective working team.

Step 2: Plan the Program Based on Needs

This step involves a detailed structure for planning a physical activity program, as discussed in the remainder of the chapter. This process begins with considering the basic elements and progresses through six action planning steps:

Basic Elements

1. Determine whom the program is for (priority group).
2. Determine with whom the program will work (change agent).
3. Determine where (context or setting) and when the program will take place.
4. Identify the physical activity behavior of interest.

Action Planning Steps

1. Learn more about the potential program participants (priority group) and the setting in which the program will take place.
2. Write down what the program seeks to accomplish: goals and objectives for the physical activity program.

3. Identify the important influences on physical activity to be changed by the program and select program strategies or activities based on these.

4. Draw or write out the logic model for how the program will work.

5. Identify resources that will be needed to carry out the physical activity program.

6. Develop a specific work plan for carrying out the program (implementation planning).

Basic Elements

The basic elements include whom the program will be for, who will work with it, what type of physical activity behavior is to be changed, and where and when the program will take place. Planners sometimes feel as though they are going in circles as they consider these basic issues—and, in fact, the process is cyclical. That is, some of these elements might need to be revisited several times before final decisions are made. For example, planners might have initially been interested in designing a club soccer team program for after-school participation by middle school students in a housing development. The planners expected to be able to use a recreation facility near the housing development. Upon checking, though, they found that this facility was not available, and there was no suitable alternative space at the housing development. The planners might then decide to reconsider earlier decisions about the type of program and whom the program is for, or they might try to determine whether additional resources are available to help find a solution. This section outlines considerations for each basic element like those in the example.

Basic Element 1: Priority Group

The first basic element involves asking the question, Whom is the program for? Consider whom the program is intended to serve, often called the priority group. Define or describe the specific group that the program hopes to serve. What are their ages? Are there boys, girls, or both? What are their ethnic backgrounds? How many young people could attend? What is the best way to reach these youths? The program could be designed to work with an entire school or a specific grade level, a community recreation agency, a faith organization, a housing development, a neighborhood, a clinic, or other groups of potential participants.

Sometimes the priority group might be determined based on where the interested professional works; for example, if the person interested in developing the intervention works in a school system, he or she thus has students as the primary audience of the program. Or, choosing the priority group might be a result of organizational priorities. For example, the person planning the program may work for the health department, which may have a strategic plan that includes working with physical education teachers. Regardless of the priority group of interest, it is helpful to describe the group in detail.

Basic Element 2: Change Agent

The second basic element involves the question, With whom will the program work? There are several groups that a program can work with or through. A program might deliver services directly to children if the program director works directly with youth or is affiliated with a group or organization that has direct access to youth such as a school, community agency, or faith organization. However, adults interested in getting youth more active often do not have direct access to youth but must gain access to them by working with another organization. In such cases, they can go through an authorizing agent or work with a change agent to gain access to young people. An authorizing agent is a member of an organization that can provide the program direct access to the population once the appropriate permissions have been granted. After contact has been authorized, program activities can be delivered directly to the priority audience through coordination with the appropriate person in the authorizing agency. For example, a Girl Scout group or faith organization might allow someone to come in and conduct a physical activity program with the children after all clearances have been obtained.

Change agents are typically adults who work in schools, community agencies, faith organizations, and other youth-serving agencies. Using this approach, program staff work directly with the change agent, usually by providing training. The change agent in turn delivers the activities of the program to the priority youth. Possible change agents include personnel or staff such as school teachers, school staff, recreation staff, and youth program leaders. When the plan includes a change agent, the first goal is to work with the change agent, who will then conduct the class or program that will change the behavior—increase the physical activity—of the youth. For example, to offer a program for students in physical education classes, program staff need to get the necessary approvals from school

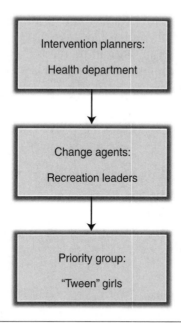

Figure 7.2 Planning flowchart.

administrators and provide program training and materials for physical education teachers. The teachers then carry out the program activities in their classes. Typical change agents for programs that seek to change physical activity in youth include teachers and coaches in school settings, staff in community agencies or organizations, youth program directors in faith organizations, and parents. Figure 7.2 graphically represents the agents and priority group in an intervention. In this example, the health department wishes to affect the physical activity behavior of 10- to 12-year-old girls and uses recreation leaders as change agents to deliver the intervention.

Basic Element 3: Time and Place

The third basic element involves where and when the program will take place. Where the program will take place might or might not be where the children are recruited. For example, a program might gain access to children for promotion purposes through a school setting but provide actual activities after school at a nearby recreation facility. Activity options for a program will be based on space, facilities, and equipment available. The following are lists of some of the settings in which physical activity programs for youth might take place. It is also important to consider when the program should be offered in terms of time of day, week, and year, as this might affect availability of both the facility and the target population.

Schools
- Physical education
- Homeroom
- Other classes (such as health education)
- Before school day begins
- During lunch or other breaks
- School facilities after school, on weekends, or during summer or other break times

Community
- Structured programs
  - Recreation center-organized activity programs: after school, weekends, and summer
  - Organized sport programs: after school, weekends, and summer
  - Church-organized programs and sports: after school, weekends, and summer
  - Summer camps
  - Fitness programs: after school, weekends, and summer
  - Instructional programs (such as dance, martial arts, self-defense): after school, weekends, and summer
- Unstructured programs
  - Recreational center: free recreational time, pickup games
  - Church: free recreational time and pickup games
  - Parks: free recreational time, walking trails, hiking, water recreation, and games
  - Community: skating parks, safe places to bicycle and skate
  - Play at home
  - Family activities and family participation in physical activity events
  - Bicycling or walking to school

Business

- Commercial skating rinks
- Fitness and health clubs with programs and activities for youth, families, or both
- Private facilities for dance, gymnastics, martial arts, and so on
- Support provided by business partners for development of safe programs or facilities in communities

Basic Element 4: Outcome

The last basic element involves the question, What are the physical activity behaviors of interest? It is important to list and describe the specific physical activity behaviors that the program seeks to influence. Action planning, which we discuss next, includes developing objectives for the physical activity program that specify what physical activity behaviors the program seeks to promote. For now, it is important to determine whether the program will focus on changing youth behavior, namely increasing physical activity or decreasing physical inactivity, or whether it will focus on an outcome related to youth behavior such as physical fitness or degree of overweight. Table 7.1 outlines questions to consider in describing the physical activity behavior that a program intends to influence.

Use Worksheet 7.2 in the appendix to summarize the basic elements and prepare for the action planning steps.

Table 7.1 Defining the Specific Physical Activity Behavior for the Program

QUESTIONS*	CONSIDERATIONS
Frequency: How often should the activity take place?	Times per day, per week, per month, or per year
Duration: How long should the activity last?	Single versus multiple bouts; accumulated activity over a day or week; amount of time in a given bout
Intensity: How difficult should the activity be?	Activities can be light, moderate, vigorous, or very vigorous
Goal: Is the goal to maintain current physical activity level or to increase physical activity level?	Maintain or increase current level of the duration, frequency, intensity, or a combination of these

(continued)

Table 7.1 *(continued)*

QUESTIONS*	CONSIDERATIONS
Activity type: What types of activities will be offered or encouraged?	Biking for transportation
	Dance
	Sports (team and individual)
	Unstructured, health-promoting activity such as walking, jogging, bicycling, swimming
	Informal structured activity such as games, pickup sports, exercise videos

*The background, experience, interests, and skill levels of the target group must be considered for all questions.

Action Planning Steps

After working through the basic elements, a planning team has a preliminary list of ideas and options. It is now time to begin a more detailed planning process using action planning steps (see the list provided at the beginning of the section on step 2). As the planning process continues, the team might revisit and change some decisions about the basic elements. By the time the team progresses through the planning steps, a specific plan for the physical activity program will be developed. Here we describe each of these planning steps in more detail.

Action Planning Step 1: Learn More

The first action planning step is to learn more about the priority group (potential participants) and the setting in which the program will take place. Intended program recipients, or priority groups, are often described in terms of such demographics as age, race, and gender or with reference to settings such as school- and community-based programs. This general description of the priority group is just a beginning. To develop effective physical activity programs, the program planners must know and understand the youth in terms of the social and cultural context in which they live and in which the program will take place.

• **Priority group.** At this point in the planning process, planners know some descriptive characteristics of the priority group. In addition to identifying needs or problems such as high levels of inactivity, planners must find out what interests and pastimes are popular with the intended audience. There are many approaches to obtaining this information, ranging from informally asking questions of a few honest youth to conducting formal needs and interests assessments using questionnaires or focus groups. By knowing the intended audience well, program planners will be able to plan a program that will be attractive to the audience of interest.

- **Change agents.** By this point in the planning, contact should have been made with the identified change agents so that their feedback can be considered and, if appropriate, incorporated into the program plan. If the project requires training change agents, such work should be scheduled through the appropriate organizational channels to provide training with minimal disruption. For example, if the change agents are teachers, their in-service training might be arranged during an event that has been previously scheduled. Program planners should establish ways to communicate regularly with change agents and their supervisors, if applicable, because regular communication will increase understanding and enhance relationship development. For instance, program planners should find out the best time and the best channel (such as telephone or e-mail) for contacting key people.

- **Context of program.** It is also necessary to consider the setting or organizational context of the program and how that will affect program implementation. For example, programs working with schools must consider the school schedule from daily, weekly, and yearly perspectives. Program planners might need to know when classes start and end, how long they last, when lunch is served, and how the daily schedule varies during the week. It is important to have a contact person within the organization or community who knows the setting and context very well.

Action Planning Step 2: Determine Goals and Objectives

Write down what the program seeks to accomplish: goal(s) and objectives for the physical activity program. Preliminary decisions about the specific physical activity behavior that the program wishes to address are reviewed at this point in the planning process. Goal(s) and measurable objective(s) for the program based on the specific program focus must now be written. A goal is usually a general statement about what the program hopes to accomplish and is not directly measurable. For example, goals for physical activity at fictional Middleburg Middle School and Middleburg High School are presented in the sidebar. Objectives are more specific than goals and should be stated in terms of the change that the program is supposed to create (e.g., change in physical activity), not in terms of what the program planners or implementers intend to do (e.g., provide a physical activity program).

Examples of Goals

- By the end of this academic year, students at Middleburg Middle School (MMS) will be physically active during their after-school time.
- By the end of this academic year, students at Middleburg High School (MHS) will engage in moderate-to-vigorous physical activity (MVPA) most days of the week.

Physical activity interventions in youth are usually designed to change physical activity behavior. Some programs might also be designed to change components of health-related fitness, such as cardiorespiratory fitness and body composition. The examples provided in this chapter focus on behavioral objectives, or the expected change in physical activity behavior in the priority group; however, objectives can be based on other measurable activity-related outcomes, including health-related fitness. See chapter 9 for more information on commonly measured outcomes in youth physical activity programs.

Objectives should also be SMART: Specific, Measurable, Achievable, Relevant, and Time Bound (U.S. Department of Health and Human Services [DHHS], 2002). For a behavioral objective, this means outlining the expected amount of change in a specific physical activity behavior that will occur in a particular group and within a specified time period. To illustrate, a national-level example taken from Healthy People 2010 (DHHS, 2000) is provided in the sidebar "Examples of SMART Objectives" and broken down into SMART parts. Also shown in the sidebar are examples of local behavioral objectives.

Examples of SMART Objectives

National Level Healthy People 2010 Objective 22-6
Increase the proportion of adolescents who engage in moderate physical activity for at least 30 minutes on five or more of the previous seven days from 27% to 35% by 2010.

Priority group: adolescents (students in grades 9-12) in the United States.

Focus of change: engage in moderate physical activity for at least 30 minutes on five or more of the previous seven days.

Change expected: increase proportion from the 1999 baseline of 27% percent to 35%.

Time frame: by 2010.

Local behavioral objective #1

Increase the proportion of 9th grade students at Middleburg High School (MHS) who engage in moderate-to-vigorous physical activity (MVPA) for at least 30 minutes on five or more of the previous seven days from 25% to 35% by the end of the program.

Priority group: ninth grade students in MHS.

Focus of change: MVPA for at least 30 minutes on five or more of the previous seven days.

Change expected: increase from 25% (2002 baseline from CDC, 2004) to 35%.

Time frame: by the end of the program year.

Local behavioral objective #2

To have 80% of all students at Middleburg Middle School (MMS) engage in moderate-to-vigorous physical activity (MVPA) after school on at least three days of the week during fall semester of current program year.

Priority group: all students in MMS (grades 6-8).

Focus of change: MVPA after school at least three days of the week.

Change expected: 80% of all students.

Time frame: by end of fall semester of current program year.

Local behavioral objective #3

The proportion of students at Middleburg Middle School (MMS) who engage in moderate-to-vigorous physical activity (MVPA) after school on at least three days of the week will increase by 25% from August to December of current program year.

Priority group: all students in MMS (grades 6-8).

Focus of change: MVPA after school at least three days of the week.

Change expected: 25% increase in proportion.

Time frame: August of current program year.

It is important that the key elements of the objective can be measured or documented. Note that objectives can be stated in terms of expected change in the target group's behavior when the preprogram or baseline level of the behavior is known. For example, since the baseline is known (27%) for the national-level objective presented in the sidebar, the expected change can be stated as a target percentage as well. Measurable objectives can also be developed if preprogram or baseline information is not known. For example, in the local objectives presented in the sidebar, expected change is stated in terms of the overall percentage of the population or an increase in proportion. However, one must know the number of students who attend MMS in order to determine how many students comprise 80%. Ways of measuring these objectives are presented in chapter 9. Worksheet 7.3 in the appendix is useful for developing SMART objectives for a program.

Action Planning Step 3: Identify Influences, Activities, and Strategies

Identify the important influences on the physical activity behavior to be changed by the program, and select activities or strategies based on those influences. The program should be designed around factors that will influence individuals to maintain a high level of activity or to become more active. In addition to the influences on individual behavior, it might be necessary to make changes to the physical environment, policies, or regulations that affect physical activity. It might be necessary to establish priorities among the influences that the program addresses if time or resources are limited—and they almost always seem to be. As described in chapter 2, there are four steps in using theory and evidence for changing physical activity behavior through a program. Use these steps to select theory-based strategies for your physical activity program. Table 7.2 (adapted from chapter 2) provides illustrations of important influences on physical activity in children and youth, as well as examples of strategies for change (Bartholomew, Parcel, Kok, & Gottlieb, 2001).

If a program has many objectives, strategies, and activities but limited resources, it might be necessary to set priorities; importance and changeability should be considered (Green & Kreuter, 1999). Give priority to strategies that have been linked to behavior change. For example, strategies that develop behavioral skills for physical activity in adolescents are more effective for promoting physical activity than are informational approaches. Changeability refers to how feasible it is for the program to make a specific behavior change. Thus, priority should be given to strategies that have been shown to be effective in changing behavior. Use

Table 7.2 Influences on Physical Activity and Strategies for Changing Physical Activity Behavior

INTENDED PURPOSE	GENERAL METHODS	EXAMPLES OF STRATEGIES
Individual		
To increase self-efficacy, behavioral capability, and behavioral skills	• Modeling or demonstration • Guided practice with feedback • Goal setting • Reinforcement	Modeling: Show videotapes of role models getting reinforced; have role models describe positive experiences through testimonials.
To increase intentions and positive expectations for physical activity	• Verbal persuasion • Modeling with vicarious reinforcement	Skill development: Facilitators demonstrate and teach skills (such as overcoming barriers and time management) in small groups; participants evaluate videotaped vignettes and practice the skill in pairs, with feedback.
Interpersonal		
To create social environments that support physical activity; to develop or enhance social support for physical activity	• Modeling with vicarious reinforcement • Creating visible social expectations • Strengthening existing networks • Creating new social networks	Social support: Teach students support-seeking skills (individual-level approach); have students choose activity buddies; involve parents directly in mother-daughter or father-son physical activity events.
Organizational		
To create organizations with policies and practices that support physical activity	• Planned organizational change	Planning group: Form committee in school that is authorized to assess and make recommended changes to policies and practices in school that affect opportunities for activity for all students.

(continued)

137

Table 7.2 (continued)

INTENDED PURPOSE	GENERAL METHODS	EXAMPLES OF STRATEGIES
Community		
To create communities and environments that provide physical activity opportunities and safe access to them	• Partnership and coalition development • Media advocacy • Policy advocacy	Partnership development: Work with several organizations toward the common goal of providing fun and accessible after-school physical activity programs for middle school youth.

Adapted from Bartholomew, Parcel, Kok, and Gottlieb, 2001.

Worksheet 7.4 in the appendix to note the relationships between important influences on physical behavior and the methods and strategies of a program. Also refer to chapter 2 for more information on constructs that can be used to help generate behavioral objectives.

Packaged physical activity programs, for which the planning has already been done, are available. Many of these programs are very effective when implemented as prescribed. However, before selecting a prepared program, planners must ensure that their priority group is similar to the one on which the program was based and that resources are available to buy sufficient material and fully carry out the program. Training is a critical component and might be overlooked when programs such as curricula are purchased. Before committing resources to purchase a prepackaged program, planners should consider trying out some of the activities to ensure a good fit with the priority population and the setting.

Action Planning Step 4: Draw the Logic Model

Draw or write the logic model for the program. A logic model lays out, in words or a diagram, how selected program strategies and methods will result in achieving the objectives for the target group. An example of a basic logic model is provided in figure 7.3. Planning proceeds from the right side of the figure to the left, beginning with the desired outcome and moving through the steps to decide what the physical activity program will do. A logic model will help you understand how the program is supposed to work and will provide an important guide for planning the program evaluation, as discussed in chapter 9.

For example, partners can work together to put on fun programs for kids, using strategies such as providing kids with activity choices, non-

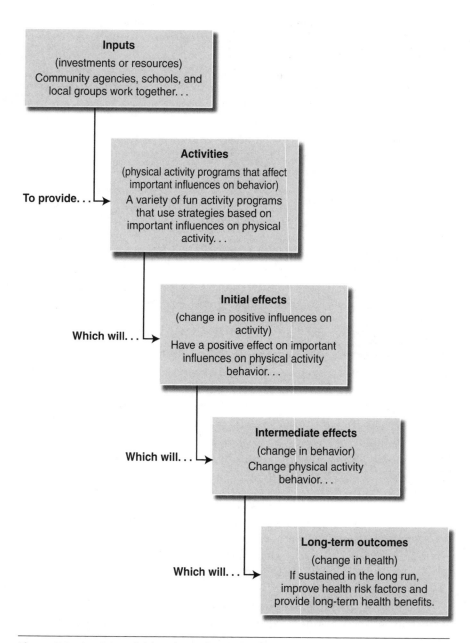

Figure 7.3 Logic model for physical activity program.

competitive and competitive options, and an emotionally safe environment that allows them to interact and enjoy themselves. Program participants will be physically active and stay with the program because they enjoy it, and they will develop confidence in their ability to be physically active and get support from friends in the program. This confidence and support should lead to ongoing engagement with physical activities and, in the long run, result in improved health outcomes such as reduced risk factors for heart disease or decreased body fat (see figure 7.3). These long-term health outcomes are usually beyond the scope of many physical activity programs because of the amount of follow-up time needed. However, the other elements of the logic model serve as a guide to how program activities are going to achieve the physical activity objectives. Worksheet 7.5 in the appendix is a useful template for developing a logic model for a physical activity program.

Because it is so easy to get lost in the details of program planning, it is helpful at this point to step back from the details of planning and describe the program in plain language using Worksheet 7.6 (see appendix).

Action Planning Step 5: Identify Resources

Identify the resources necessary for carrying out the physical activity program. All programs require resources, including appropriately trained staff, space, and perhaps equipment, depending on the program requirements. Significant funds are usually needed to hire and pay staff and to obtain and maintain appropriate space. Of course, it is also possible to conduct some program activities using volunteers rather than paid staff, and to obtain space and equipment at little or no cost through collaboration with other organizations. Planners must remember, though, that volunteers might need training and that training also requires resources. Schools and community agencies may have facilities and skilled staff for physical activity programs, but organizational priorities, staff availability, and competing programs may make it difficult to provide accessible programs. Other resources that might be needed for physical activity programs targeting youth include transportation and incentives for participation.

There are a variety of ways to obtain resources for physical activity programs. Organizations or groups might be able to put on programs within existing budgets, especially if providing physical activity programming is part of the organizational mission, such as that of a recreation center, or from special allocations of funds. Alternatively, a proposal can be developed and submitted to appropriate local, state, or federal funding sources. Assistance with grant writing might be obtained from local colleges, universities, and some nonprofit organizations. Other fund-raising strategies include approaching groups, organizations, or businesses for funds and equipment and working cooperatively with other groups or organizations that can provide in-kind resources such as staff or space.

An important resource consideration, particularly for new programs, concerns infrastructure needs. Infrastructure includes the following elements:

- Organizational structure that specifies lines of authority and communication
- Defined procedures within an organization or group for planning and carrying out programs
- Defined roles for staff and others involved in planning and carrying out the program
- Procedures for how priorities are set and decisions made for the group or organization
- Procedures for managing funds
- Skilled or trained staff
- Space, facilities, and equipment
- Mechanism to promote programs and recruit participants
- Mechanism to monitor programs and safety

The following is a list of resources by category that might be required to implement a program. Also see chapters 9 and 10 for a discussion of items that need to be considered when evaluating and monitoring a physical activity program.

- Staff
  - Ensure linkages to program plan (Worksheets 7.2 through 7.6)
  - Promote program and recruit participants
  - Handle program registration (if applicable)
  - Coordinate program logistics (identify program leaders, coordinate space and equipment, deal with barriers such as transportation)
  - Lead physical activity programs (will leaders need training?)
  - Oversee provision of physical activity programs
  - Consider volunteers, as appropriate

- Materials
  - For program promotion and participant recruitment, including parent information
  - For program registration
  - Instructional materials (if applicable)
- Equipment and supplies
  - Physical activity equipment
  - Refreshments (if applicable)
  - Computer equipment and Internet access (for records and communication)
  - Office and other supplies
- Facility and space
  - Scheduling
  - Costs
  - Sharing agreements
- Transportation (if applicable)
- Incentives (if applicable)

Action Planning Step 6: Develop a Specific Plan

The next step is to develop a specific work plan for carrying out the program. In this final step, the details of "who does what when" are spelled out. This step will ensure that the elements needed to make the program operational are in place and that responsible individuals know what they are supposed to do and when they are supposed to do it. The details of this action step are listed in Worksheet 7.7 in the appendix, which can be used to identify the specific activity to be implemented, the person who will be responsible, and the date by which the task should be completed.

SUMMARY

It is essential to identify and involve stakeholders in planning physical activity programs for youth. Begin program planning by identifying the basic elements of the program: who, what, when, and where. After preliminary decisions have been made, there are six action planning steps to guide the development of a detailed plan for the program: (1) Learn more about the potential program participants and the setting in which the program will take place; (2) write down what the program seeks to accomplish—goals and objectives for the physical activity program; (3) identify the important influences on physical activity to be changed by the program and select program strategies or activities based on them; (4) draw or write out the logic model for how the program will work; (5) identify resources that will be needed to carry out the physical activity program; and (6) develop a specific work plan for carrying out the program.

As noted earlier, program planning and evaluation planning should be accomplished at the same time. This chapter covered program planning; for evaluation planning, please continue with chapters 9 and 10, which present further detail about focusing the evaluation of the physical activity program.

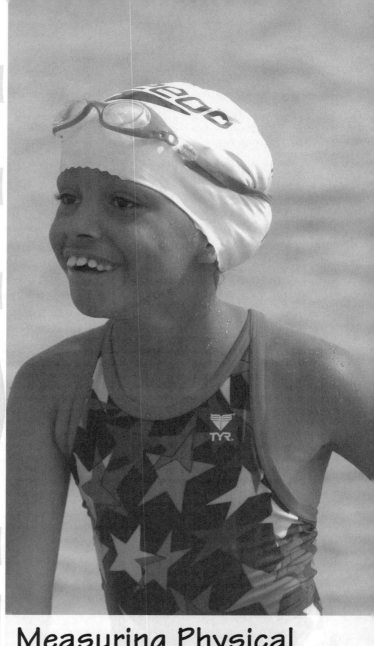

EIGHT

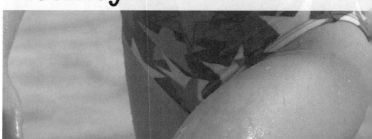

Measuring Physical Activity

Previous chapters have emphasized the importance of systematically evaluating the effectiveness of interventions to promote physical activity in children and youth. Regardless of the setting in which interventions are implemented, the overarching goal of such programs is usually to enhance young people's health or fitness, or both, by increasing their levels of physical activity. An extensive body of scientific evidence documents that increasing physical activity typically produces improvements in indicators of health and fitness. But the fact that physical activity can improve health and fitness does not prove that a particular intervention actually has produced important changes in health or fitness. For that matter, without careful evaluation, we cannot be sure that an intervention has produced the desired overall increase in physical activity in a target group, or even that the program has been carried out in the way intended. Therefore, a comprehensive protocol for evaluation of a physical activity intervention requires measuring physical activity as well as the health or fitness variables that are expected to be affected by the anticipated increase in physical activity. A primary purpose of this chapter is to present methods for measurement of physical activity in children and youth. In addition, the chapter provides an overview of measures of important influences on physical activity and an overview of the available measures for two key outcome variables, physical fitness and body composition, that are often targeted by physical activity interventions.

Public health researchers have defined the term physical activity in a broad, inclusive manner to refer to any muscle-powered movement. Physical activity in children and youth includes walking to school and running in physical education class, performing household chores and shooting baskets in the driveway, playing actively with siblings and competing on a soccer team. Because young people can be physically active in so many different ways, measurement of physical activity in a valid manner is not as simple a process as it might seem.

Measurement of physical activity is complicated not only by the fact that activity comes in many specific forms but also by the fact that it is performed in myriad settings, for widely varying periods of time, and at intensities ranging from very light to extremely vigorous. Researchers have developed a substantial number of methods for measuring physical activity. Some of these methods provide only a global, overall measure of a child's physical activity level, while others provide very detailed indicators of physical activity performed at various intensities, for various periods of time, in various settings, and in various modes. The following sections provide an overview of the accepted methods for measurement of physical activity in young people. More detailed reviews of these methods are available in other sources (Sirard & Pate, 2001; Pate & Sirard, 2000). Table 8.1 presents an overview of methods that are often used to measure physical activity in children and youth. Only the most commonly used methods are discussed in the following sections.

Table 8.1 Measures of Physical Activity in Youth

MEASURE	OBJECTIVITY	STRENGTHS	LIMITATIONS
Subjective measures			
Self-report	Low	Can be used in large studies	Recall errors; survey must be validated; young children cannot recall accurately
Interview	Low	Can be used in large studies	Requires trained interviewers; bias; recall errors
Proxy report	Low	Adults can report for young children	Low validity; recall errors
Diary	Low	Fairly accurate, identifies activity patterns	Subject burden; subject reaction
Objective measures			
Doubly labeled water	High	Very accurate, physiological marker, criterion measure	Expensive; high subject burden; not appropriate for population studies; cannot identify activity patterns
Direct observation	High	Accurate, can identify activity patterns	Extensive observer training; subjects may react; not appropriate for population studies
Heart rate	High	Physiological marker, accurate at the group level	Influenced by environment and diet; subject compliance

(continued)

Table 8.1 *(continued)*

MEASURE	OBJECTIVITY	STRENGTHS	LIMITATIONS
Objective measures *(continued)*			
Accelerometers	High	Objective, identifies patterns of activity	Do not detect all types of movements; subject compliance
Pedometers	High	Objective	Cannot identify activity patterns; subject compliance

Adapted from Pate and Sirard, 2000.

Subjective Measures of Physical Activity

As indicated in table 8.1, physical activity can be measured both subjectively and objectively. Whereas objective measures often employ an external device such as a pedometer to identify levels of physical activity, subjective measures must rely on an individual's recall of events and truth in reporting. Measures such as self-reported activity patterns often cannot be used in studies that target young children because of their inability to recall past events accurately (Pate & Sirard, 2000). However, subjective measures like interviews and participant questionnaires can often be more effectively used in large studies than costly measures such as those that use pedometers or accelerometers. In this section, we present some subjective measurement techniques that have been used successfully in physical activity interventions involving children and adolescents.

Self-Report Measures

Self-reported measures of physical activity were used most often in the past because they are noninvasive and simple to administer. However, young children are too limited in recall and other cognitive abilities to provide useful self-reports of their participation in physical activity. Children and youth over the age of 10 are able to provide reasonably reliable and valid self-reports of their activity participation. In general, children do well with procedures that depend on recalling physical activity for only the previous two to three days, and they seem to do better with recalling their participation in specific forms of activity such as basketball or dancing than with reporting the length of time they engaged in certain activities. Like adults, children are able to recall and report structured, vigorous activities much better than they can report informal, moderate-intensity activities. The following are brief descriptions of the self-report measures of physical activity that have been most widely used with young people.

Previous Day Physical Activity Recall (PDPAR)

The Previous Day Physical Activity Recall, reproduced in appendix 8.A, requires the respondent to recall the dominant activity he engaged in during a series of 30-minute time increments on the previous day (Weston, Petosa, & Pate, 1997). For each activity reported, the child provides a rating of the intensity with which he recalls engaging in the activity. For example, a child might recall that the dominant activity engaged in during the 3 to 3:30 p.m. time block was soccer. The child would consult a menu of activities provided with the instrument, select the number corresponding to soccer, enter it for the 3 to 3:30 p.m. time block, and then provide an intensity rating to describe how vigorously he recalls engaging in the activity. A series of graphics is provided to guide the child in selecting an appropriate intensity rating. This same pattern is followed for each 30-minute time block.

The data collected with PDPAR are reduced through assigning an intensity rating, or MET value, to each 30-minute time block. The MET is a unit representing the intensity of physical activity in terms of the multiple of resting metabolic rate that is typically associated with performance of that activity; for example, jogging might require about 6 METs, meaning that energy expenditure during jogging is six times greater than resting energy expenditure. This process uses data from the scientific literature to rate the intensity of various activities as adjusted by the child's own rating of intensity. Table 8.2 lists and defines various physical activities, intensities, and MET levels common in children and youth. For example, soccer performed at an intensity rated as "hard" would be assigned a MET value of 7. The child's overall physical activity for a fraction of a single day (e.g., 3:00-6:00 p.m.), a complete day, or a series of days can be scored in two ways: as the average of all MET values assigned for the reported activities, or through determination of the number of 30-minute time blocks for which activities were reported with MET values about selected cut points (e.g., blocks of vigorous activity with values of 6 METs or greater).

Table 8.2   Physical Activity Levels

ACTIVITY LEVEL	DEFINITION	EXAMPLES
Sedentary	1.0 METs	Lying down, sitting, watching television
Light	1.1 METs-2.9 METs	Walking at 2 mph, slow cycling, stretching or light conditioning exercises
Moderate	3.0 METs-5.9 METs	Walking at 3-4.5 mph, cycling at 5-9 mph, doubles tennis
Vigorous	6.0 METs-8.9 METs	Walking at >5.0 mph, jogging, cycling at ≥10 mph or uphill, singles tennis
Very vigorous	≥9.0 METs	Running

The PDPAR methodology has been shown to be most effective when used as a series of one-day recalls, preferably for five to seven consecutive days. However, it has also been used as a three-day recall instrument in which each of the previous three days is recalled in a single session. This modification of the instrument, known as 3DPAR, has been validated for use with children age 12 and older (Pate, Ross, Dowda, Trost, & Sirard, 2003).

Self-Administered Physical Activity Checklist (SAPAC)

Another widely used instrument for self-reported measurement of physical activity in youth is SAPAC (Sallis, Buono, Roby, Micale, & Nelson, 1993; Sallis et al., 1996). This instrument, which is supplied in appendix 8.B, contains a list of 21 common forms of exercise, sport, and play. The respondent indicates each of those activities that was performed on the previous day during each of three time blocks: before school, during school, and after school. For any activity that was performed, the respondent estimates the amount of time she engaged in that activity during the specified time block. The data on the form can be reduced in several different ways to create indices that reflect the child's physical activity on the reported day. The number of activities reported can be totaled, the number of minutes of activity reported can be calculated, or total "MET-minutes" can be determined through application of a rating of exercise intensity to each reported form of physical activity. SAPAC forms can be completed as a series of one-day recalls of previous days, or reports for several preceding days can be completed in one session.

The composite of at least three and up to seven days of SAPAC reports is required to generate an index that reflects "typical" or "usual" physical activity behavior.

A number of other procedures for measuring physical activity by self-report in children and youth have been developed. A summary can be found in the work of Sallis and Saelens (2000).

Surrogate Reports of Physical Activity in Children

It is also possible to estimate physical activity in children by collecting information from the adults who supervise them. Parents and teachers who observe children during much of their day can provide useful ratings of the activity levels of those children. This technique is particularly useful with young children who cannot report their own activity and in situations in which objective measures of activity are not feasible. Some studies have shown that parents overestimate their children's activity (Noland, Danner, DeWalt, McFadden, & Kotchen, 1990), but others indicate that parents' reports correlate well with children's physical fitness (Murphy, Alpert, Christman, & Willey, 1988). Global ratings have often been used for these reports (e.g., "On a scale of one to five, relative to other children his/her age, how physically active is your child?"). More detailed systems have been developed as well. Manios and colleagues (1998), for example, developed a system in which teachers reported the physical activity levels of 6-year-old children during free play periods and parents reported the physical activity levels of the same children during after-school hours and on weekends. Heart rate monitoring was used to evaluate the proxy report measures, both of which were found to be useful for assessing moderate-to-vigorous physical activity in young children.

Objective Measures of Physical Activity

In recent years, new measures of physical activity have been developed in an attempt to overcome some of the limitations of self-report measures. Objective measurement techniques avoid the biases and recall limitations that are characteristic of children. While objective measures are not without limitations, these new approaches do appear to provide very useful information. Objective measures of physical activity come in two primary forms: direct observation and electromechanical monitors (pedometers and accelerometers). In this section we provide brief introductions to these methods.

Direct Observation of Children's Physical Activity

Several systems have been developed for structured recording of physical activity in children. Some focus on observation of children in specific settings, such as physical education classes, playgrounds, or preschools. Most of these systems use a similar procedure for observing and recording the level of physical activity. The Children's Activity Rating Scale (CARS) (Puhl, Greaves, Hoyt, & Baranowski, 1990) or modifications thereof can be used to score a child's activity level using a five-point scale in which 1 refers to sedentary and 5 corresponds to vigorous, whole-body movement. Because young children tend to be active in short spurts, "instantaneous" observation periods are usually employed. For example, if the physical activity level of a group of children in a playground setting were to be measured, an observer might randomly select five children for observation during a 30-minute period. During each 15-second period, the observer might focus on one of the five children, observe her activity level for 5 seconds, and then take 10 seconds to record the observed level of activity on paper or in electronic form. The group's overall activity would be the composite of the 120 observations recorded during the 30-minute period; 24 observations would have been made on each of the five selected children. Table 8.3 lists and briefly describes several of the direct observation systems that have been used to measure physical activity in young people.

Pedometry

Because such a large percentage of the typical child's overall physical activity comes in the form of walking, running, or other kinds of bipedal locomotion (e.g., skipping, jumping, leaping), step counting can be used to measure children's physical activity. Pedometers are small, battery-powered mechanical devices that count steps. They come in many styles and models, but most are relatively inexpensive (less than $25). Pedometry has limited utility as a research measure of physical activity because children tend to react to the monitor and can easily manipulate it. However, because pedometers have been shown to provide reasonably

Table 8.3   Direct Observation Systems for Recording Physical Activity

OBSERVATION SYSTEM	REFERENCE	DESCRIPTION
Children's Activity Rating Scale (CARS)	DuRant et al. (1993) Puhl et al. (1990)	Records minute-by-minute observations of young children's physical activity levels; can be used in a variety of settings.
Observation System for Recording Activity in Children–Preschool (OSRAC-P)	Trost et al. (2003) Dowda et al. (2004) Brown et al. (2006)	Designed to determine the physical activity level of children in preschools and to identify related environmental factors. Focal child system; assesses activity level, activity type, physical environment, and social environment.
Behaviors of Eating and Activity for Children's Health: Evaluation System (BEACHES)	McKenzie et al. (1991)	Designed to simultaneously code physical activity, eating behaviors, and related environmental factors. Focal child system; used in a variety of settings.
System for Observing Play and Leisure Activity in Youth (SOPLAY) System for Observing Fitness Instruction Time (SOFIT) System for Observing Play and Recreation in Communities (SOPARC)	McKenzie et al. (2000) McKenzie et al. (1991) McKenzie et al. (2006)	Collects observational data on the number of children and their activity levels within a specified area. Uses systematic scans of children and environmental factors within the area.

valid indices of overall physical activity and are relatively inexpensive, they have been used to provide feedback to children in activity interventions. Extensive information on pedometers is available in other sources (Tudor-Locke et al., 2004; Tudor-Locke, Williams, Reis, & Pluto, 2002; Tudor-Locke & Bassett, 2004).

Accelerometry

Accelerometers are electromechanical devices that are sensitive to movement (see figure 8.1). They are small, beeper-size instruments that are usually worn on a belt at the waist. These devices record "activity counts" that reflect the intensity of movement on an instantaneous basis.

The counts are stored on a computer chip in time increments that can be determined by the user. When accelerometers are used with children, activity counts are often stored in 15- or 30-second increments, but shorter or longer increments can be used. Data can be stored for several days; and for observation of usual physical activity, it is desirable for the person to wear the monitor for a full week. Accelerometry has become state of the art for measurement of physical activity in research studies. Because accelerometers are quite expensive ($400 or more per unit), however, they have not come into wide use as adjuncts in physical activity interventions. An important advantage to accelerometry is that these instruments can be calibrated in a manner that allows the determination of activity intensity on a time unit basis. For example, across a day of monitoring, the minutes spent in moderate, vigorous, or very vigorous physical activity can be ascertained. Although accelerometry is an important advance in measurement of physical activity, the method does have limitations. It is important to note that accelerometers measure only physical activity and provide no information on the type of physical activity performed or the physical or social setting in which the activity was undertaken. For best practices on the use of accelerometers, see the study by Ward and colleagues (2005).

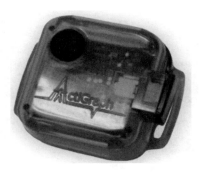

Figure 8.1 Actigraph accelerometer.

Influences on Physical Activity

In chapter 2, we identified a number of important influences on physical activity. Many physical activity programs target change in these influences, as well as in physical activity behavior. If a program seeks to change an influence on physical activity, it might be important to measure that influence. In this section, we describe approaches to measuring three of the most commonly identified influences on physical activity behavior in children and adolescents: perceived self-efficacy, social support, and enjoyment.

Perceived self-efficacy for physical activity is an individual's belief in his ability to be physically active even if he encounters a variety of barriers.

Perceived self-efficacy is consistently related to participation in physical activity in youth. Refer to chapter 2 for a more complete discussion of this issue. Instruments to assess perceived self-efficacy typically ask the respondent to rate the confidence that she or he has to be active in the presence of specific barriers to physical activity. See appendix 8.C for an example of a physical activity self-efficacy scale used with children and adolescents.

Enjoyment of physical activity is also consistently related to young people's participation in physical activity. It stands to reason that youth who do not enjoy an activity will not continue to participate in it. See appendix 8.D for an example of a scale used with children and adolescents that measures enjoyment of physical activity.

Social support for physical activity from adults is important for youth, especially since in most cases youth need adult assistance to participate in physical activity opportunities. Young people usually cannot pay fees, purchase needed equipment, or provide their own transportation and thus rely on parents or caregivers for support. Social support from peers has also been shown to be important, particularly for adolescents. Instruments used to measure social support for physical activity in youth usually include items that address different kinds of support from family and peers. See appendix 8.E for an example of a social support scale used with children and adolescents.

Physical Fitness Measures

"Physical fitness" has been defined in many ways, but fundamentally this term refers to a person's ability to perform physical activity. Because physical activity comes in many different types and is performed at various intensities and in numerous settings, physical fitness is operationally defined in multidimensional terms. In its broadest sense, physical fitness encompasses the ability to perform activities as different as the 50-meter dash and the marathon. Table 8.4 lists the components of physical fitness, defined (Pate, 1988) as sport-related and health-related physical fitness. Sport-related physical fitness components are associated with sport or athletic performance. Health-related components have been linked to one or more health outcomes. Because this book focuses on physical activity interventions that are designed to promote health, we limit the discussion to measures of the physical fitness components that are health related. Further, this section primarily addresses measures of

Table 8.4 Components of Physical Fitness: Sport-Related and Health-Related

COMPONENT	DEFINITION*
Sport-related physical fitness	
Muscular power	The ability to release maximum muscular force in the shortest time
Speed	The ability to perform a movement within a short period of time
Agility	The ability to rapidly change the position of the entire body with speed and accuracy
Balance	The maintenance of equilibrium in a stationary position or during moving
Coordination	The ability to use the senses together with body parts in performing motor tasks
Health-related physical fitness	
Cardiorespiratory fitness	The ability of the circulatory and respiratory systems to supply oxygen during sustained physical activity
Body composition	The relative amounts of muscle, fat, bone, and other vital parts of the body
Muscular strength	The ability of the muscle to exert force during an activity
Muscular endurance	The ability of the muscle to perform without fatigue
Flexibility	The range of motion available at a joint

*U.S. Department of Health and Human Services (1996).

Adapted from U.S. Department of Health and Human Services, 1996.

fitness that can be used in nonlaboratory settings such as schools and community fitness centers.

Cardiorespiratory Fitness

Cardiorespiratory fitness, one's ability to perform prolonged whole-body activity, is sometimes seen as the single most important reflection of overall physical fitness. This component of fitness has a critical impact on a person's ability to perform many occupational and leisure tasks and is known to be related to several key chronic diseases, such as coronary heart disease and type 2 diabetes. Persons with good levels of cardiorespiratory fitness are able to perform demanding work and leisure tasks without excessive fatigue and have a reduced risk of developing chronic diseases.

Since cardiorespiratory fitness has such overriding significance, many measures of this fitness component have been developed for use in laboratory, quasi-laboratory, and field settings. The "gold standard" measure of cardiorespiratory fitness is maximal aerobic power or $\dot{V}O_2$max, the maximal rate at which a person is able to consume oxygen during exhaustive exercise (see figure 1.2 in chapter 1). This oxygen consumption capacity is the major physiological determinant of one's ability to sustain vigorous whole-body activity like jogging or cycling. While $\dot{V}O_2$max is a very precise and reliable measure, the test is expensive and time-consuming and requires performance of exhaustive exercise. Because of these limitations, the $\dot{V}O_2$max test is rarely used in applied settings. Numerous field tests of cardiorespiratory fitness have been developed through validation against $\dot{V}O_2$max. In the following sections, we provide brief descriptions of several of the most commonly used field tests of cardiorespiratory fitness.

Physical Working Capacity-170

Persons with higher levels of cardiorespiratory fitness, as compared with their less fit counterparts, manifest lower heart rates at any given exercise intensity. Accordingly, the heart rate response to graded endurance exercise can be used to measure cardiorespiratory fitness. Several different test protocols have been developed on the basis of this phenomenon. One of the most commonly used is the Physical Working Capacity-170 (PWC-170) test. This test is administered using a bicycle ergometer, which is adjusted to three or more progressively increasing rates of effort. As shown in figure 8.2, heart rate increases steadily as effort on the cycle is increased. The heart rate response is plotted against effort on the cycle (i.e., power output), and the effort associated with a heart rate of 170 beats per minute is estimated. The greater the power output at a heart rate of 170, the higher the cardiorespiratory fitness. The PWC-170 has two advantages: It is non-weight bearing so that heavy participants are not penalized; and the test is submaximal, meaning that it does not require an exhaustive effort. However, the test does require a laboratory-grade cycle ergometer.

20-Meter Shuttle Run

The 20-meter shuttle run (22 yards; also known as the PACER Test) has come into wide use in recent years as a means of measuring cardiorespiratory fitness in physical education classes and comparable settings (Liu, Plowman, & Looney, 1992). Minimal equipment is required, and the test can be administered on an open, flat, safe surface that is at least 25 to 30 meters

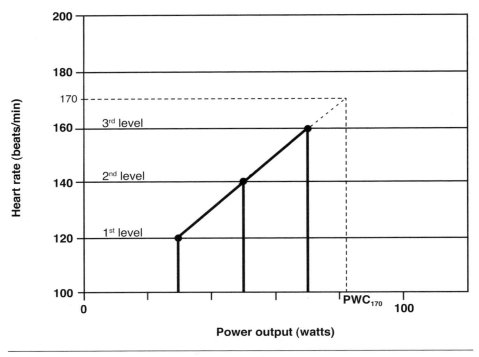

Figure 8.2   Physical Working Capacity-170 graph.

(27-33 yards) in length (see figure 8.3). A gymnasium is preferred if large numbers of children are to be tested at once, but a hallway can be used to test individual participants. The test procedure involves the child's running back and forth between two lines that are 20 meters apart. The running pace is gradually increased as the participant is required to keep up with an auditory signal that occurs at an incrementally increasing rate. Children continue running until they can no longer keep up with the signal. The number of laps completed can be used to estimate cardiorespiratory fitness expressed as $\dot{V}O_2max$ (milliliters of oxygen consumed per kilogram body weight per minute). The 20-meter shuttle run has the advantage of being a task that most children and youth seem to enjoy, but it does require maximal effort.

Distance Runs

Both time-limited (e.g., distance run in 12 minutes) and distance-limited (e.g., time to run 1 mile or 1.6 kilometers) runs have been shown to provide valid estimates of cardiorespiratory fitness in children and youth.

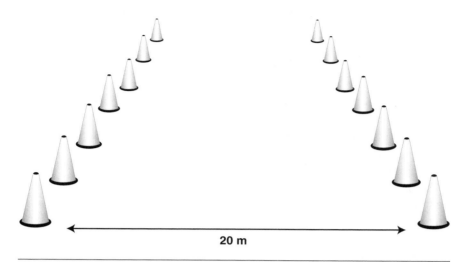

Figure 8.3 The 20-meter shuttle run.

These tests have been used extensively since the 1960s, and experience indicates that they are acceptable if the participants are fully oriented to the test and have acquired a reasonable sense of appropriate pacing. However, these tests do require maximal effort, and they are often not found to be enjoyable by young people. Table 8.5 provides brief descriptions and references for the most widely used distance running tests of cardiorespiratory fitness.

Table 8.5 Running Tests Used to Evaluate Physical Fitness

TEST	CRITERION	REFERENCES
600-yard run-walk	Time required to run-walk 600 yards	Doolittle & Bigbee (1968) Metz & Alexander (1970) Safrit (1973)
1-mile run-walk	Time required to run-walk 1 mile	Wiley & Shaver (1972)
9-minute run-walk	Distance covered in 9-minute walk-run	Jackson & Coleman (1976)
12-minute run-walk	Distance covered in 12-minute walk-run	Doolittle & Bigbee (1968) Maksud & Coutts (1971) Jackson & Coleman (1976)

Body Composition

Body composition refers to the percentage of a person's total body weight that is accounted for by adipose or fat tissue (% body fat). Body composition is considered a component of health-related physical fitness because a person's fatness influences his ability to perform many types of physical activity, and body fatness is known to be powerfully influenced by physical activity habits. Hence it is often of interest to measure body composition as a factor that might be influenced by physical activity interventions.

Many measures of body composition have been developed, and the best measures provide quite precise estimates of % body fat. These methods include hydrostatic weighing (measuring a person's weight on land and during submersion under water) and dual-beam X-ray absorptiometry (DEXA), which uses very low-dose X rays to differentiate between the body's fat and lean tissues. While both of these methods have been widely used in research studies, neither is suitable for field-based research in health promotion programs because of the cost and participant burden involved. Fortunately, there are several measures of body composition that are suitable for use with large numbers of participants and in field settings. These include weight-to-height ratios such as the body mass index (BMI) and various anthropometric techniques that involve measures of one or more skinfold thicknesses.

Body Mass Index

Body mass index is a mathematical ratio between body weight and height (BMI = weight in kilograms / height in meters^2). Body mass index has come into wide use as a measure of weight status that can be applied in large, population-based studies. It is an attractive measure of body composition because it requires measurement of only height and weight. However, one should note that BMI can provide erroneous information on weight status in some individuals. For example, those who perform a great deal of resistance exercise and experience a large gain in lean weight might show a high BMI but not be excessively fat. With that limitation, BMI is a low-cost and convenient measure of body composition that is now being extensively used in public health, medical, and educational settings.

Because of growth and developmental issues, BMI is used differently with children and adolescents. BMI for children, also known as BMI-for-age, is used to determine if children are underweight, at risk of overweight, or overweight. Because body fat changes as children grow and develop, each of these categories is based on a percentile rather than a specific BMI. Table 8.6 presents BMI-for-age categories.

Growth charts developed by the Centers for Disease Control and Prevention are used to determine a child's percentile based on age and sex (CDC, 2000). A specific BMI value might place different children in different weight categories. For example, a girl with a BMI of 22 would be in the 95th percentile at age 9, but in the 75th percentile at age 14. Table 8.7 provides another example of BMI changing over time while percentile stays the same (National Center for Chronic Disease Prevention and Health Promotion, 2004).

Skinfold-Based Anthropometric Measures

Body fat is stored subcutaneously, or under the skin, as well as around the organs in the abdominal cavity and other sites in the body. The thickness of a person's skinfolds, which include the top two layers of the skin and the underlying fat tissue, is related to the overall percentage of the body weight that is fat. Because measurement of skinfold thicknesses is a relatively inexpensive and unobtrusive procedure, many methods for estimating body fatness from skinfold thicknesses have been developed for both adults and children. One well-validated and widely accepted

Table 8.6 BMI-for-Age Categories

WEIGHT CATEGORY	BMI-FOR-AGE
Underweight	<5th percentile
At risk of overweight	≥85th to <95th percentile
Overweight	≥95th percentile

Table 8.7 Example of BMI-for-Age and BMI Percentile for a Boy From Age 2 to Age 13

AGE	BMI	BMI-FOR-AGE PERCENTILE
2	19.3	95th
4	17.8	95th
9	21.0	95th
13	25.1	95th

procedure is the one used by FITNESSGRAM. With this procedure, a physical education teacher, fitness leader, or other trained adult uses skinfold calipers to take two skinfold measures, one at the triceps of the right arm and one at the right calf. The two measurements are summed, and the total is converted to percent body fat using charts provided in the FITNESSGRAM Test Administration Manual (Cooper Institute for Aerobics Research [CIAR], 1999). For example, a boy with a summed skinfold measure of 21 millimeters has approximately 16.4% body fat. A girl with a summed skinfold measure of 31 millimeters has approximately 24% body fat. Although skinfold measures are inexpensive, it is important to note that the validity of these procedures requires the measures to be taken in a highly standardized manner. Accordingly, those who administer these measures must be appropriately trained and experienced.

Muscular Strength and Muscular Endurance

Muscular strength refers to the maximum force that a person can exert by contracting a specified muscle group. Muscular endurance is the ability to perform repeated contractions of a specified muscle group against substantial resistance. For example, in the forearm curl movement depicted in figure 8.4, an expression of muscular strength would be the greatest weight that a person could move through the full range of motion one time or the 1-repetition maximum (1RM). In contrast, a measure of muscular endurance would be the maximum number of times a person could perform that movement against a resistance corresponding to 50% of the 1RM. Muscular strength and endurance are important to day-to-day functions because they determine a person's ability to perform tasks that require overcoming significant resistances such as lifting heavy objects or carrying a child. These components of fitness are important to health because muscular strength in the abdomen and trunk is a key factor in prevention of low back pain, one of the most common and costly health problems in contemporary society.

In field settings, muscular strength and endurance can be measured using free weights or a supported-weight system. Muscle strength and endurance are specific to each muscle group; for example, a person can have strong legs and weak abdominal muscles. Although muscular strength and muscular endurance are related components, they are not identical. Accordingly, a series of tests is needed to determine muscular strength and muscular endurance for key muscle groups. In administra-

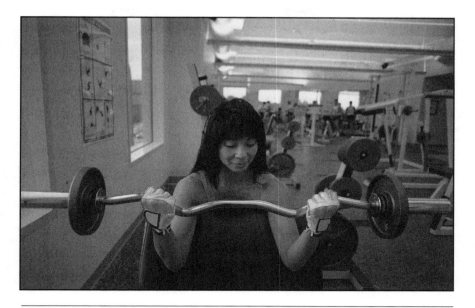

Figure 8.4 Forearm curl.

tion of these tests, safety is an overarching concern. Participants should be carefully instructed in the proper lifting procedure and should be closely spotted while performing the movements. These tests have been used successfully with children, even children of elementary school age, but considerable caution should be taken in the use of these procedures with young children.

In practice settings such as physical education classes, muscular endurance can be measured using calisthenic exercises in which body weight is the resistance moved. Common examples of these tests are the sit-up, push-up, and pull-up tests. These tests provide reasonably valid measures of muscular endurance if they are administered with proper standardization and if the participants are strong enough to perform the movements at least several times. Because resistance is provided by the person's body weight, these tests provide measures of relative muscular endurance. Clearly, a heavier child is required to move more weight than a lighter child. The maximum number of repetitions of a movement performed therefore indicates the person's ability to work against his or her own body weight. Detailed procedures for administration of these tests are provided elsewhere (CIAR, 1999).

Flexibility

Flexibility is the maximum range of motion possible in a joint or a series of joints. For example, a youth's ability to reach toward his or her toes is determined by the flexibility at the hip joint, which in turn is determined in large part by the extensibility of the muscles and other tissues in the lower back and hamstring areas. Flexibility is an important determinant of one's ability to perform certain physical tasks, including many sport skills. Good flexibility is thought to reduce the risk of injury during performance of vigorous exercise, and maintenance of good flexibility in the low back region is an important factor in prevention of low back pain.

As with muscular strength, flexibility is specific to each joint. In children and youth, flexibility is most commonly measured for the low back and hamstring areas. A number of different tests of low back flexibility have been developed for use with youngsters in field settings. Figure 8.5 depicts a flexibility test that can be used in physical education classes and other fitness settings.

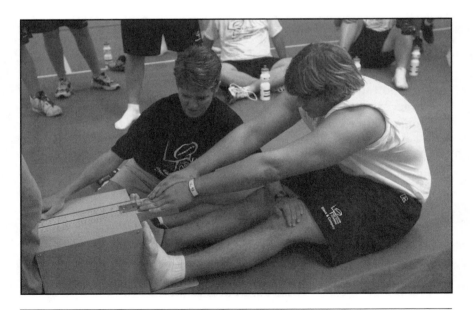

Figure 8.5 Flexibility test.

SUMMARY

Measuring physical activity in children and youth is a complex process. Many aspects of physical activity, including frequency, intensity, duration, mode, and setting, can be measured or studied. Some measurement tools provide a global measure of a child's activity, while others assess activity in a particular setting or at a particular time. Some tools are appropriate for use in large population studies, while others must be used in a clinical setting. Still others measure factors related to physical activity, such as cardiorespiratory fitness or BMI. The scientist or health professional who plans to measure physical activity in children or youth must have a clear objective in mind and select measurement tools appropriate to achieving that objective. The need to increase physical activity levels in children and youth is clear. Equally clear is the need to accompany all physical activity interventions with appropriate methods of measuring physical activity and related factors in order to identify the interventions that are most likely to improve the health and fitness of children and youth.

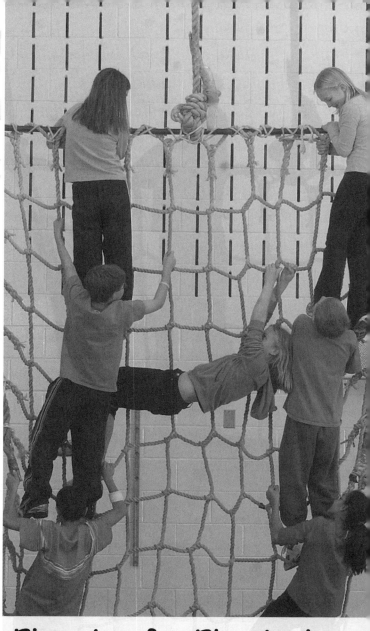

NINE

Planning for Physical Activity Program Evaluation

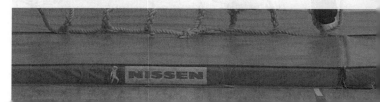

The primary aim of any evaluation effort is to make improvements in programs. Program evaluation is one of the most thorough ways to determine how well an intervention has succeeded and to provide feedback for subsequent implementation. Although program evaluation is conducted in a systematic manner and is analytical in nature, it is not the same as research (see sidebar). Program evaluation can be used to analyze a program's structure, activities, organization, and social and political environment. It can assess how well a project has achieved its goals and objectives, and it can also measure the costs and impacts in order to indicate where improvements can be made (Fink, 1993). In addition to providing useful information for program implementers and stakeholders, program evaluation can be used for the following purposes (U.S. Department of Health and Human Services [DHHS], 2002):

- To share with other communities what does and does not work
- To build community capacity and engage communities
- To influence policy makers and sources of funding
- To ensure funding and sustainability

How Evaluation Differs From Research

Evaluation

- is controlled by stakeholders (interested parties);
- involves standards of usefulness, feasibility, accuracy, and fairness;
- assesses merit, worth, and importance;
- is holistic and flexible;
- is ongoing, broad, and integrative; and
- is used to develop program capacity.

(U.S. DHHS, 2002)

Two central uses of program evaluation are (1) to assess a program's effectiveness and (2) to monitor and document program activities. The current chapter explains the use of effectiveness evaluation for physical activity programs in examining the impact of the program on outcomes such as physical activity levels or physical fitness. Chapter 8 presented approaches for measuring common outcomes of physical activity programs, including physical activity and fitness. Planning for program monitoring is described in chapter 10.

As noted in chapter 7, planning the program and planning its evaluation are part of the same process. Planning steps 1 and 2 were covered in chapter 7 (see review in figure 9.1). Step 3, evaluating the effectiveness

Planning phase

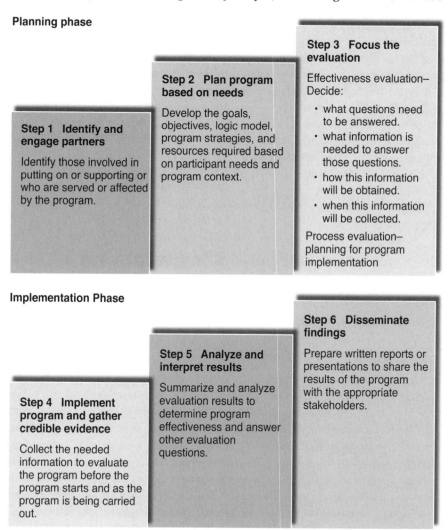

Step 3 Focus the evaluation

Effectiveness evaluation–Decide:

- what questions need to be answered.
- what information is needed to answer those questions.
- how this information will be obtained.
- when this information will be collected.

Process evaluation–planning for program implementation

Step 2 Plan program based on needs

Develop the goals, objectives, logic model, program strategies, and resources required based on participant needs and program context.

Step 1 Identify and engage partners

Identify those involved in putting on or supporting or who are served or affected by the program.

Implementation Phase

Step 6 Disseminate findings

Prepare written reports or presentations to share the results of the program with the appropriate stakeholders.

Step 5 Analyze and interpret results

Summarize and analyze evaluation results to determine program effectiveness and answer other evaluation questions.

Step 4 Implement program and gather credible evidence

Collect the needed information to evaluate the program before the program starts and as the program is being carried out.

Figure 9.1 Planning and implementing physical activity programs.

Adapted from the Centers for Disease Control and Prevention (CDC), 1999, and U.S. Department of Health and Human Services, 2002.

of the program, is the primary topic of this chapter. Chapter 10 covers process evaluation planning for monitoring program implementation (step 3) and program implementation itself (steps 4-6).

Review of Program Planning

In step 1, identifying and engaging partners, stakeholders are identified and involved in program planning (see chapter 7). Stakeholders should remain involved throughout the program planning, implementation, and evaluation process. A stakeholder might be a representative of the school district, an employee at the work site, or a member of the community.

In step 2, planning the program based on needs, the program plan is developed, including goals and objectives, theory- and evidence-based methods and strategies, a logic model, resources required, and a plan for program implementation (see chapter 7).

Evaluation planning (step 3), the topic of this chapter, extends this planning effort and evolves from the SMART objectives, methods, and strategies based on important influences on physical activity and on the logic model.

Step 3: Focus the Evaluation

Nine elements of a plan for program effectiveness evaluation are described briefly in table 9.1. The remainder of this chapter presents a more detailed description of each of the elements.

Evaluation Purposes

It is important to work with stakeholders to discuss the approach that will be taken to evaluate the effectiveness of the intervention and the ways in which this information will be used. Program effectiveness evaluation can focus on short-term or long-term impacts or outcomes. A common short-term objective of a physical activity program is change in physical activity behavior. An example of a long-term objective is change in a health outcome such as risk factors related to heart disease. Program effectiveness evaluation compares the results of the program to an objective or a standard to measure the extent to which the program was successful. If the program has measurable objectives, evaluating program effectiveness is fairly straightforward—a matter of finding out whether or not the objectives were met. If there are no objectives or other standards to

Table 9.1 Program Effectiveness Evaluation Elements

ELEMENT	DESCRIPTION
1. Evaluation purposes	How the effectiveness evaluation will be used
2. Evaluation questions	Questions the effectiveness evaluation should answer; usually based on SMART objectives
3. Evaluation design	Timing of data collection; use of comparison group(s)
4. Sampling	How members of the target group will be identified to be surveyed, interviewed, observed
5. Data sources, data collection tools, and methods	Where the information comes from that is needed to answer the evaluation questions; what instruments or tools should be used to collect evaluation information
6. Data collection procedures	The plan for data collection
7. Data entry, analysis, and summary	Methods used to enter and summarize or analyze data to answer evaluation questions
8. Plan for using results	How findings will be used and shared with stakeholders
9. Resources needed	Resources needed to conduct the evaluation

use, a standard must be determined from such reliable sources as the Physical Activity Evaluation Handbook (DHHS, 2002).

Evaluation Questions

As noted earlier, effectiveness evaluation focuses on what effects the program had or the extent to which SMART objectives were met. Consider again the Middleburg Middle School (MMS) after-school program and the objective for this program presented in chapter 7 and in the sidebar. The primary effectiveness evaluation question is, "Did the MMS after-school program accomplish the primary objective?"

SMART Objective for the MMS After-School Program

To have 80% of all students at MMS engage in 30 minutes of moderate-to-vigorous physical activity (MVPA) after school on at least three days of the week during the current program year.

As illustrated in the SMART objective, the expected result is an increase in MVPA after school, so specific effectiveness evaluation questions are as follows:

- Did 80% of all students at MMS engage in 30 minutes of MVPA after school on at least three days of the week during fall semester?
- How many of the students at MMS engaged in 30 minutes of MVPA after school on at least three days of the week during fall semester?

The program logic model might also suggest questions that relate to the effectiveness of the program. For example, the logic model indicates that there should be an increase in physical activity enjoyment, self-efficacy, and social support (see table 9.2). Therefore, additional evaluation questions include the following:

Behavior Change
- What effect did program participation have on participants' self-efficacy for physical activity?
- What effect did program participation have on participants' enjoyment of physical activity (not enjoyment of the program itself)?

Influences on Behavior
- What effect did program participation have on participants' social support for physical activity from friends?
- What effect did program participation have on participants' social support for physical activity from family (parent or guardian)?

Use Worksheet 9.1 in the appendix to summarize the effectiveness evaluation questions (changes in behavior and influences on behavior) for your program based on the SMART objectives and the logic model.

Evaluation Design

Program effectiveness evaluation is designed to answer the question, "Were the observed effects the result of the physical activity program or of some other factors?" Two aspects of program evaluation design can be considered to help answer this question: (1) the groups involved in the evaluation and how these groups are formed and (2) the timing of evaluation data collection.

Groups Involved

At the minimum, there must be one group involved in the evaluation: participants in the program. A stronger design involves at least two

Table 9.2 Logic Model for the MMS After-School Program

INPUTS	ACTIVITIES	INITIAL EFFECTS	INTERMEDIATE EFFECTS	LONG-TERM OUTCOMES
Investments or resources	Physical activity programs that target important influences	Change in important influences	Change in physical activity behavior	Change in health outcomes
Community agencies, schools, and local groups work together to . . .	provide a variety of fun activity programs that use strategies based on important influences (e.g., enjoyment, perceived self-efficacy, and social support) on physical activity, which . . .	will have a positive effect on important influences on physical activity behavior (e.g., enjoyment, perceived self-efficacy, and social support), which . . .	will change physical activity behavior (e.g., MVPA after school), which . . .	will, if sustained in the long run, improve health risk factors and provide long-term health benefits.

groups, one receiving the physical activities of the program (also known as the intervention group) and one that is not receiving activities of the program (also known as a control or comparison group). Members of the control or comparison group might receive no program activities at all, or they might receive a different set of activities that should not affect their physical activity behavior. The advantages of having a comparison group are discussed in more detail later in the chapter.

How these groups are formed is also important. Interventions using groups formed from individuals who volunteer to be in the program or through use of a preexisting group such as a youth club are considered to have weaker designs. In contrast, groups formed through random placement of potential participants into the intervention or comparison group are considered stronger designs. We discuss this issue further in a later section.

Timing of Data Collection

Evaluation data can be collected before, during, and after the program (see figure 9.2). Typical times to collect evaluation data are before the program is implemented (baseline or pretest data collection) and imme-

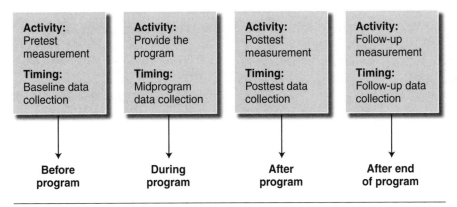

Activity: Pretest measurement	**Activity:** Provide the program	**Activity:** Posttest measurement	**Activity:** Follow-up measurement
Timing: Baseline data collection	**Timing:** Midprogram data collection	**Timing:** Posttest data collection	**Timing:** Follow-up data collection
Before program	**During program**	**After program**	**After end of program**

Figure 9.2 Timing of data collection for effectiveness evaluation.

diately after the program is implemented (posttest data collection). Sometimes data are collected during the program (midprogram data collection) and again at some later time after the program has ended (follow-up data collection). While it is possible and often simpler to collect only posttest data, stronger evaluation designs call for data to be collected before and after the program. Follow-up data collection, some time after the program has ended, might be appropriate if one of the evaluation objectives focused on maintaining changed behavior over time. Data collection during the program might be appropriate if the program is sufficiently long, if there is a well-defined use for such interim information based on SMART objectives, and if resources are available to conduct this kind of data collection.

Design of Alternative Explanations for Program Results

The purpose of a careful evaluation design is to help rule out alternative explanations for the results obtained after the program. For example, suppose that measures taken at the end of a physical activity program show that 90% of program participants are meeting recommendations, and the objective was for at least 80% of the target group to meet them. Does this mean that the program was a success? Not necessarily! Program evaluation includes considering alternative explanations for this result. A one-group, posttest-only design does not rule out other possible explanations for this result, including the following:

- No pretest assessment: The participants were already active at the beginning of the program, but their activity at that time was not measured.
- Maturation: Natural physical or cognitive development in the program group resulted in improved outcomes apart from the program.
- History: The statewide physical education organization was also promoting physical activity after school during this time.
- Selection: The participants who volunteered for the program were more motivated than typical students.
- Attrition: The participants who were not active dropped out earlier and were not measured at posttest.

Addition of a pretest assessment to the one-group design makes it possible to assess change in the program. However, there are still alternative explanations for program results, including the following:

- Maturation, History, Selection, Attrition
- Testing: By taking the pretest, participants were able to score better at posttest.
- Instrumentation: The pretest and posttest instruments were not the same or were not given in the same way.
- Statistical regression: Participants had very low or very high scores at the beginning.

Having a group that is comparable to the program or intervention group can help rule out alternative explanations such as maturation, history, and testing, since the groups should be affected equally. Having participants randomly assigned to groups reduces the effects of selection. Using trained staff and having consistent measurement procedures will reduce instrumentation problems. The problem of attrition must be addressed as a part of getting and keeping participants in the program through overcoming barriers to participation.

Table 9.3 describes the most common program evaluation designs and the ways in which they help reduce such alternative explanations for observed effects. This information demonstrates that it is best to have a pretest and a posttest, and to have a group that is comparable to the intervention group. For additional information on evaluation design, see the book by Shadish and colleagues (2002).

Table 9.3 Common Evaluation Designs for Assessing Program Effectiveness

DESIGN	UNLIKELY EXPLANATIONS	POSSIBLE EXPLANATIONS
Posttest only; one group	Cannot evaluate change at all, much less change due to the program	
Pre- and posttest; one group		Maturation History Selection bias Attrition Testing Instrumentation Statistical regression
Pre- and posttest; two groups, formed by "convenience" (quasi-experimental)	Maturation History Testing	Instrumentation Statistical regression Selection bias Attrition
Pre- and posttest; two groups, formed by random assignment (experimental)	Maturation History Testing Selection bias	Instrumentation Statistical regression Attrition

Adapted from U.S. Department of Health and Human Services, 2002.

Other considerations for evaluation design include length of the program, availability of statistical expertise, feasibility, and resources available to perform the evaluation.

Sampling

Sampling involves determining how members of the priority group(s) will be selected to participate in data collection, including surveys, interviews, or observations. Making decisions about sampling includes answering the following questions: (1) How many people will be included? (2) How will the people be selected? In addition, these issues must be considered:

- SMART objective, which often defines the priority population
- Size of the priority population (do you include everyone, or a sample?)

- Subgroups of the priority population (e.g., males and females)
- Budget and time constraints

For example, since the MMS after-school physical activity SMART objective is based on change in the entire MMS student population, the simple sampling option of measuring the activity of only those who participate in the program will not answer the evaluation question. It is also necessary to know the total number of students at MMS in order to answer this evaluation question. Similarly, if the intervention targets subgroups, such as students by grade level or sex, it is necessary to design sampling that will ensure enough participants in each category. If the total number of students at MMS is small, surveying everyone can be considered. However, if the number is large, the number surveyed as part of evaluation is often set by budget, other resources, and access to the population. If everyone cannot be surveyed, then an appropriate sampling strategy must be devised. Common among such strategies are convenience sampling, simple random sampling, and stratified random sampling, detailed in table 9.4.

Table 9.4 Approaches to Sampling in Program Evaluation

TYPE	DESCRIPTION	COMMENTS
Convenience	Those surveyed are selected based on accessibility or convenience—for example, the participants that volunteer to be in a program.	With this type of sample, you must interpret evaluation results carefully, mainly because groups of individuals chosen this way are likely to be different from the whole population in important ways. Also, the sample will not be representative of the population.
Simple random	Using a simple technique like a random numbers table, individuals surveyed are chosen from the priority population.	This is one approach to obtaining a sample that is representative of the priority population based on statistical theory.
Stratified random	The priority population is split into strata (such as males and females or by grade level), and those surveyed are selected randomly from each stratum.	This approach ensures that you select enough individuals in specific subgroups to be able to make conclusions about how the program affected them.

Table 9.5   Approaches to Sampling for Evaluating the MMS After-School Physical Activity Program

TYPE	DESCRIPTION	COMMENTS
Convenience	The survey is administered to the after-school physical activity program participants.	This sampling strategy could provide useful evaluation information, although the makeup of the group will likely differ from the population of students in the school (e.g., they may be more motivated), limiting confidence in claims about the effectiveness of the physical activity program.
Simple random	Using a computer program (available through the school district) to make the selection, the survey is given to a random sample of all students at MMS.	This is an effective sampling strategy to assess how the program affected the entire population; it will be difficult to show results if few students at MMS participate in the after-school program.
Stratified random	Using a computerized program available through the school district to make the selection, the survey is given to equal numbers of male and female students from grades 6 and 7 at MMS.	This is an effective sampling strategy to assess how the program affected males and females in grades 6 and 7; similar to the situation with the simple random sampling approach, it will be difficult to show results if few males or females in these grades at MMS participate in the after-school program.

Table 9.5 illustrates these three sampling approaches with the MMS after-school program example. A school population is fairly well defined compared to populations in community settings. If a high level of scientific confidence or assistance with defining the population is needed, consider identifying an expert in statistics or biostatistics from a health department or local college or university who can develop your sampling plan.

Use Worksheet 9.2 in the appendix to summarize the evaluation design and sampling plan for your physical activity program. A separate worksheet for each of the program's evaluation questions might be needed, as not all evaluation questions will be answered with the same design.

Data Sources and Data Collection Tools

A comprehensive approach to physical activity program evaluation requires measuring physical activity as well as the variables (health, fitness, or both) that are expected to be affected by the anticipated increase in physical activity. For this element of the plan, you must identify the information needed to answer each evaluation question, including the sources of this information and the tools that will be used to gather it. It can be very time-consuming and labor intensive to develop good tools to assess behavior or influences on behavior. It is also difficult to develop good measures from scratch. Therefore, it is often preferable to use tools and procedures that have been tested in other programs. It is always a good idea to pilot test the tools you have selected with a small number of youth from the priority group, for example by giving them the survey and asking for feedback about what is clear and unclear to them. In chapter 8, we presented an overview of the available measures for key variables that are often targeted by physical activity interventions. These variables include physical activity, physical fitness, body composition, and selected psychosocial factors. Table 9.6 summarizes key physical activity variables and

Table 9.6 Data Collection Tools for Evaluating Effectiveness of Physical Activity Programs and Influences on Physical Activity Behavior

EVALUATION QUESTION (VARIABLE)	SOURCE OF DATA	POSSIBLE DATA COLLECTION APPROACHES	EXAMPLES
Physical activity	Program participants	Self-reported measures	PDPAR, 3DPAR SAPAC
		Objective measures	Direct observation (CARS, OSRAC-P) Pedometry Accelerometry
	Adults involved with program participants	Surrogate measures	Parent or teacher report
Physical fitness	Program participants	Cardiorespiratory fitness	PWC-170 20-meter shuttle run Distance runs
		Body composition	Body mass index Skinfold anthropometric

(continued)

Table 9.6 *(continued)*

EVALUATION QUESTION (VARIABLE)	SOURCE OF DATA	POSSIBLE DATA COLLECTION APPROACHES	EXAMPLES
Perceived self-efficacy	Program participants	Self-report	Self-efficacy scale
Perceived social support	Program participants	Self-report	Social support scale
Enjoyment	Program participants	Self-report	Enjoyment scale

measures identified in chapter 8 that have been used for evaluating the effectiveness of physical activity programs in children and adolescents. Refer to chapter 8 for additional information on tools available to evaluate your physical activity program.

For example, the objectives for the MMS after-school physical activity program suggest the types of measures that might be appropriate. Because the main objective pertains to MVPA, a measure of physical activity is needed. Given the limited resources available for the project and the setting, a self-report instrument is selected: 3DPAR, the 3-Day Physical Activity Recall detailed in chapter 8. The influences on activity that are targeted in this program are cognitive in nature, so self-report tools are needed to measure such variables as enjoyment, self-efficacy, and social support that cannot be directly observed. Table 9.7 provides examples of data collection tools and data sources suggested by the specific evaluation questions for the MMS after-school physical activity program.

Use Worksheet 9.3 in the appendix to summarize the selection of data sources and data collection tools.

Data Collection Procedures Plan

Data collection procedures describe the logistics of data collection. They include planning and describing details of the steps for collecting data on schedule. After data sources have been identified, data collection tools and methods have been identified and pilot tested, and the design has been determined, the following checklist of procedures should be considered.

Table 9.7 **Examples of Data Sources and Data Collection Tools Suggested by the Evaluation Questions for the MMS After-School Physical Activity Program**

DATA SOURCES	DATA COLLECTION METHODS AND TOOLS
Did 80% of all students at MMS engage in 30 minutes of MVPA after school on at least 3 days of the week during fall semester?	
School records Students in school	Physical activity survey for all students in school: 3DPAR
What effect did program participation have on participants' self-efficacy for physical activity?	
Program participants	Self-efficacy questionnaire (written survey)
What effect did program participation have on participants' social support for physical activity from friends?	
Program participants	Social support questionnaire (written survey)
What effect did program participation have on participants' social support for physical activity from family?	
Program participants' parents	Social support questionnaire (written survey)
What effect did program participation have on participants' enjoyment of physical activity?	
Program participants	Enjoyment questionnaire (written survey)

Checklist of Data Collection Procedures

1. Sufficient number of staff are available to collect data.

2. Sufficient numbers of data collection tools are available when needed.

3. Instructions about how to administer the tools are written down.

4. Data collectors are trained to administer the instruments consistently.

5. Permissions or notifications required for collecting data have been obtained.

6. Data collectors check completed instruments for missing or invalid information.

7. Completed instruments are delivered to the appropriate person for data entry, analysis, and summary.

8. Staff roles for various data collection tasks are clearly defined.

Data Entry and Analysis or Summary

The data entry and analysis part of the plan describes how data will be handled and summarized after they are collected, and how data will be handled if not entered into a computer software program. The plan includes what kind of analysis or summary will be used to answer the evaluation questions, with the goal of getting data into a form that can be summarized and interpreted. Elements of the plan include coding of the data, data entry/software, and analysis or summary of the data. Effectiveness evaluation data are usually quantitative, as shown in table 9.8. The data analysis approach should be selected based on what it takes to answer the evaluation questions. Seek assistance for accomplishing data entry and analysis as needed. If none of the planning partners has this expertise, identify experts from the health department or a local college or university. See the summary of coding, data entry, and data

Table 9.8 **Approaches to Coding, Data Entry, and Analysis or Summary for Quantitative Data**

PROCESS	EXPLANATION
Coding	Coding is typically numeric. Some instruments are "self-coding" in that the respondent circles, selects, or writes down a number. For nominal data, the numeric codes may be assigned at this stage (e.g., 1 = male and 2 = female).
Software	Free software: EpiInfo (available at http://www.cdc.gov/epiinfo) Database packages such as Access and Excel Statistical software packages such as SPSS and SAS
Data entry	Indirect data entry: Previously collected data are coded; then an operator enters the data into a computer using software. Direct data entry: Data are entered into a computer at the time of data collection; for example, computer-assisted telephone interviewing and Internet surveys.
PROCESS	EXPLANATION
Analysis or summary	Descriptive analysis summarizes important characteristics of the group surveyed (such as age, sex, grade level) using frequencies, means, ranges, and so on. Answering evaluation questions may involve statistical analysis such as t-tests, analysis of variance, and chi squares to determine change from pre- to posttest and to compare intervention and control groups.

Adapted from U.S. Department of Health and Human Services, 2002, and The Health Communication Unit, 1997.

analysis for the effectiveness evaluation questions in the example of the MMS after-school physical activity program.

Plan for Coding, Data Entry, and Data Analysis or Summary for the MMS After-School Physical Activity Program

Evaluation Question 1

Did 80% of all students at MMS engage in MVPA after school on at least three days of the week during fall semester?

Coding: Questionnaire data collected from all students before and after program.

Data entry/Software: Codes entered into computer by data entry operator using EpiInfo.

Data analysis/Summary: Calculate percent of students meeting PA recommendation posttest after considering pretest levels; number of blocks of MVPA during after-school hours on 3DPAR.

Evaluation Question 2

What effect did program participation have on participants' self-efficacy for physical activity?

Coding: Questionnaire data collected from all students before and after program.

Data entry/Software: Codes entered into computer by data entry operator using EpiInfo.

Data analysis/Summary: Calculate change in self-efficacy score from pre- to posttest and test for statistical significance.

Evaluation Question 3

What effect did program participation have on participants' social support for physical activity from friends?

Coding: Questionnaire data collected from all students before and after program.

Data entry/Software: Codes entered into computer by data entry operator using EpiInfo.

Data analysis/Summary: Calculate change in social support score from pre- to posttest and test for statistical significance.

Evaluation Question 4

What effect did program participation have on participants' social support for physical activity from family (parent or guardian)?

Coding: Questionnaire data collected from all students before and after program.

Data entry/Software: Codes entered into computer by data entry operator using EpiInfo.

Data analysis/Summary: Calculate change in social support score from pre- to posttest and test for statistical significance.

Evaluation Question 5

What effect did program participation have on participants' enjoyment of physical activity (not of the program itself)?

Coding: Questionnaire data collected from all students before and after program.

Data entry/Software: Codes entered into computer by data entry operator using EpiInfo.

Data analysis/Summary: Calculate change in enjoyment scores from pre- to posttest and test for statistical significance.

Use Worksheet 9.4 in the appendix to develop a plan for coding, data entry, and data analysis or summary for your program.

Plan for Using Results

It is important to outline your plan for sharing results of the program evaluation with stakeholders by answering the following questions:

- When and how will effectiveness evaluation results be shared with staff?
- When and how will effectiveness evaluation results be shared with program participants and secondary audiences?
- When and how will effectiveness evaluation results be shared with other stakeholders, including funding and sponsoring organizations?
- What is the most appropriate channel (e.g., mailing, newsletters, personal contacts, media, Web sites) and format (e.g., summary of methods and results, detailed report with tables and charts, strengths and weaknesses of the program and evaluation, recommendations) for sharing results with each stakeholder group?

Resources Required for Planning and Conducting the Program Evaluation

In this step, resources that will be required to plan and carry out the program evaluation must be identified. It is important to determine what can be accomplished with existing resources, including staff availability, staff expertise, available computers and software, funding, and available outside resources. Options for outside resources include students and faculty from colleges and universities who might be willing to assist with or without financial compensation, personnel from such state and local agencies as health departments, and paid consultants or experts.

The Centers for Disease Control and Prevention estimate that 10% of a program's budget should be spent on evaluation efforts. For example, if a pedometer challenge at the Boys & Girls Club costs $3000, then $300 should be designated for evaluation of the program's effectiveness. See the summary of resources that may be required to evaluate a physical activity program. Note that the need for many of the resources listed will depend on the specifics of the individual program.

Summary of Considerations and Resources That May Be Needed for Evaluating a Physical Activity Program

Staff or Consultant Expertise

- For evaluation design, sampling, analysis, and measurement
- For coordination of measurement and data-related activities for effectiveness evaluation
- For instrument identification or development
- For recruitment and obtaining parent permission
- For data collection
- For data entry and analysis
- For interpreting and reporting results

Materials

- Materials for recruiting participants, including parent information and permission
- Data collection tools (surveys)

185

Equipment and Supplies

- Equipment for fitness testing, monitoring physical activity, and taking other physical measures as appropriate
- Computer equipment and Internet access for records and communication
- Software for data entry and analysis
- Office and other supplies

Facility and Space Requirements

- Scheduling and costs
- Space with privacy for data collection

Transportation

Incentives

Other

It is helpful to have a written summary of the program effectiveness evaluation plan. Use Worksheet 9.5 in the appendix to summarize the overall effectiveness evaluation plan.

Finally, it is important to develop a detailed work plan (see Worksheet 9.6 in the appendix) that spells out who does what when. These steps ensure that the elements needed for the effectiveness evaluation are in place and that responsible individuals know what they are supposed to do and when they are supposed to do it.

SUMMARY

The evaluation plan to determine the effectiveness of a physical activity program for children and youth is a continuation of the program planning process. Evaluation questions, data collection tools, and data sources are ideally based on the program's objectives. Other important considerations include selection measures, sampling, evaluation design, data entry and analysis, and ways in which the results will be used. It is also important to identify and obtain the resources needed to carry out the evaluation and to develop a work plan so that tasks are carried out in a timely manner.

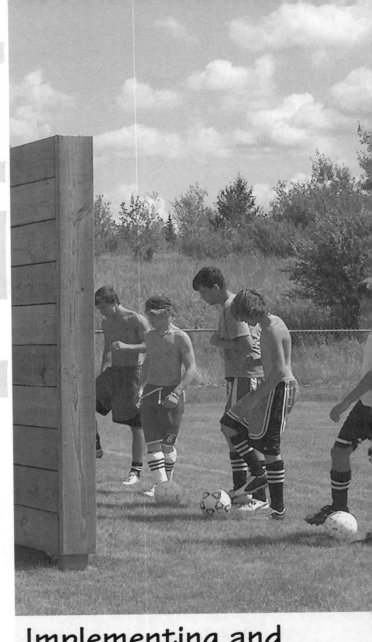

TEN

Implementing and Monitoring Physical Activity Programs

In chapters 7 and 9, we discussed planning your physical activity program (steps 1 and 2) and planning for measuring program effectiveness (step 3) (see figure 10.1). The last part of step 3 in the planning process is to monitor the program as it is carried out in order to ensure successful program implementation. Successful program implementation depends

Planning phase

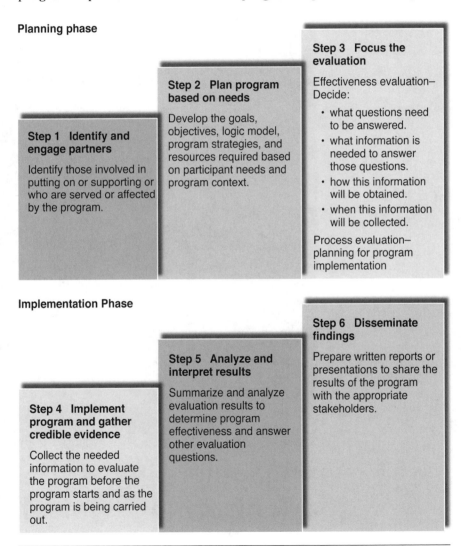

Step 1   Identify and engage partners

Identify those involved in putting on or supporting or who are served or affected by the program.

Step 2   Plan program based on needs

Develop the goals, objectives, logic model, program strategies, and resources required based on participant needs and program context.

Step 3   Focus the evaluation

Effectiveness evaluation–Decide:

- what questions need to be answered.
- what information is needed to answer those questions.
- how this information will be obtained.
- when this information will be collected.

Process evaluation–planning for program implementation

Implementation Phase

Step 4   Implement program and gather credible evidence

Collect the needed information to evaluate the program before the program starts and as the program is being carried out.

Step 5   Analyze and interpret results

Summarize and analyze evaluation results to determine program effectiveness and answer other evaluation questions.

Step 6   Disseminate findings

Prepare written reports or presentations to share the results of the program with the appropriate stakeholders.

Figure 10.1   Planning and implementing physical activity programs.

Adapted from the Centers for Disease Control and Prevention (CDC), 1999, and U.S. Department of Health and Human Services, 2002.

on monitoring throughout the process, and successful implementation will increase the likelihood of program effectiveness. This chapter covers process evaluation as well as the implementation phase (steps 4-6) of the physical activity program.

Process Evaluation Elements

Many reasons can contribute to a program's lack of effectiveness in reaching its objectives. Three possible reasons are that (1) the program was not implemented at all, (2) it was implemented differently than planned, or (3) it did not reach sufficient numbers of the target audience. Process evaluation, which involves systematic monitoring and documenting of program activities, can provide explanations for successful or unsuccessful results for a program (Bartholomew, Parcel, Kok, & Gottlieb, 2001). In the previous chapter, we presented nine elements necessary for program effectiveness evaluation. These elements, however, are equally important to take into account when one is planning the process evaluation, which is the last part of focusing the evaluation (step 3). These elements are listed again in table 10.1 and are used to illustrate how to

Table 10.1 Process Evaluation Elements

ELEMENT	DESCRIPTION
1. Evaluation purposes	How the effectiveness evaluation will be used: formative or summative process evaluation
2. Evaluation questions	Questions the process evaluation should answer; usually based on the components of the process evaluation plan
3. Evaluation design	Timing of data collection
4. Data sources, sampling, and data collection tools	Source of the information needed to answer evaluation questions; how the members of the priority group will be selected for participation in data collection; the instruments or tools to be used to collect data
5. Data collection procedures	The plan for data collection
6. Data entry, analysis, and summary	How data will be entered and summarized or analyzed
7. Plan for using results	How findings will be used and shared with stakeholders
8. Resources needed	Resources needed to conduct the process evaluation

develop a process evaluation plan to monitor the implementation of a physical activity program.

Evaluation Purposes

Always work with stakeholders to determine the important purposes of the process evaluation. Process evaluation can be used for monitoring (or formative) purposes and for documenting or judging (or summative) purposes. Process evaluation can be used to provide day-to-day monitoring of the intervention and to ensure that activities are taking place as planned and with the expected level of participation (formative use). Problems or barriers that are identified can be corrected early. Process evaluation used at the end of the intervention (summative use) provides an assessment of the success of the program implementation and seeks to explain why the program was or was not successful. In contrast, effectiveness evaluation (discussed in chapter 9) measures whether or not the program was successful in meeting its objectives (Bartholomew et al., 2001).

Six components of process evaluation apply to both monitoring and assessing program implementation: (1) the quality of the program (fidelity); (2) the completeness of the program (dose delivered); (3) the reach of the program into the priority population; (4) the amount of the program received by participants (dose received), including participant satisfaction; (5) the procedures for and barriers to participant recruitment and participation; and (6) program influences from the larger environment (context) (Steckler & Linnan, 2002; Baranowski & Stables, 2000; Saunders, Evans, & Joshi, 2006). Definitions and examples of these process evaluation elements are provided in table 10.2.

Evaluation Questions

As stated earlier, process evaluation emphasizes what is happening in the program and how well what is happening fits with the original plan. Therefore, process evaluation questions should be based on a detailed understanding of the program and how it is supposed to work from the planner's perspective. For the purposes of illustration, the Middleburg Middle School (MMS) after-school physical activity program is described in the sidebar on page 192.

There are many possible process evaluation questions, depending on the exact purpose of the process evaluation. It is imperative to select the

Table 10.2 Components of a Process Evaluation Plan

COMPONENT	DEFINITION	EXAMPLES OF QUESTIONS
Fidelity	Extent to which intervention was implemented as planned or consistently with theory and philosophy	To what extent were program strategies, such as small, enduring groups, used to increase social interaction among youth in an activity program?
Dose delivered	Amount or number of intended units of each intervention or component delivered or provided by interventionists	To what extent were all planned sessions and all components of each session (such as warm-up, activity time, cool-down, and skill building) carried out?
Reach	Proportion of the intended target audience that participated in the intervention; often measured by attendance	How many members of the target population received the program?
Dose received	Extent to which participants engaged in recommended activities and were satisfied with the program and interactions with staff, investigators, or both	How satisfied were after-school program participants with the physical activity options provided?
Recruitment	Procedures used to recruit and keep participants in the program	How were participants invited to the program? Document recruitment efforts such as number of flyers distributed at what sources, when and where announcements were made, and so on.
Program context	Aspects of the larger environment that may affect participation or program outcome	What were the effects of local and state campaigns to promote physical activity?

Adapted from Steckler and Linnan, 2002, and Baranowski and Stables, 2000.

most important questions for a given program rather than attempting to ask all possible questions. Priority questions should be selected with the input of stakeholders. Applying the six components of process evaluation to the MMS after-school physical activity program example, we can generate several potential process evaluation questions as detailed in table 10.3.

Use Worksheet 10.1 in the appendix to summarize the purposes and process evaluation questions for your program.

The MMS After-School Physical Activity Program

The after-school program will meet two days per week after school (3:30-5:50 p.m.) for six weeks. Ninety minutes are devoted to a physically active game or an activity including 45 minutes of moderate-to-vigorous physical activity. The activity component begins with a warm-up and ends with a cool-down. The activities are to include a variety of lifetime activities and cooperative games, in addition to modified sport activities. The goal is to keep all participants engaged, physically active, and having fun. The final 30 minutes are devoted to developing skills to become and remain physically active, including the following skills: communication, support seeking, goal setting, and self-monitoring.

Table 10.3 Examples of Potential Process Evaluation Questions

COMPONENT	POTENTIAL QUESTIONS
Fidelity	• Is the program being delivered as planned? If not, why not? • Are the staff leading the program in the style intended (e.g., emphasizing having fun over winning)? If not, what can be done? • Are program participants having fun? Are their friends participating in the program?
Dose delivered	• Are all sessions being offered as planned (e.g., 12 sessions total)? • Are all sessions being offered on the planned schedule? • Are all components of the sessions being provided (e.g., warm-up, activity, cool-down, and skill building)?
Reach	• How many young people are participating? Is this the expected number? If not, what are possible reasons for low participation? • What is attendance over time? Is it changing or stable? What factors are related to changes in attendance?
Dose received	• How are participants responding to the physical activity options? • How are participants responding to the way the program is operated? • What do participants like and not like about being in the program? • Are participants having fun?
Recruitment	• Are participants being recruited as planned? If not, why not? • Is transportation a barrier to participation? If so, how can it be addressed? • What are other barriers to participation? How can they be addressed?

COMPONENT	POTENTIAL QUESTIONS
Program context	• Are there other competing programs or activities? How can these be addressed in a cooperative manner?
	• What programs or initiatives similar to this one are promoting physical activity?

Evaluation Design

Evaluation design does not apply to process evaluation in the same way it applies to effectiveness evaluation. Process evaluation focuses on program implementation and therefore does not require a control or comparison group. However, when a comparison group is available, one possible use of the process evaluation is to monitor for competing programs, historical events, and other contextual factors that can affect program outcomes. In this case, process evaluation data collection should be done in both intervention and comparison groups. Also, data collection is often ongoing in process evaluation, rather than limited to time periods such as pre- and posttest data collection.

The timing of process evaluation data collection is important and will depend on the purpose of the process evaluation and the process evaluation questions. For monitoring and corrective feedback (formative) purposes, process evaluation information must be collected and fed back to program staff quickly and regularly. For summarizing overall implementation success (summative) purposes, process evaluation information might be collected less frequently. See table 10.4 for illustrations of timing the process evaluation data collection for formative and summative purposes.

Use Worksheet 10.2 in the appendix to summarize process evaluation planning for timing of data collection.

Data Sources, Sampling, Data Collection Tools, and Methods

Next we must identify the information that will be needed to answer the process evaluation questions, including the sources of this information and how members of the target group will be identified. Some general sources of information for program evaluation include people, documents, and observations (U.S. Department of Health and Human Services, 2002).

Table 10.4 Timing of Process Evaluation Data Collection

TIMING FOR FORMATIVE PURPOSES	TIMING FOR SUMMATIVE PURPOSES
Is the program being delivered as planned?	
Collect information at the end of each session to provide immediate feedback and to take corrective action, if needed.	Complete a checklist for at least four of the 12 sessions each semester; summarize program fidelity by semester.
Are all sessions being offered on the planned schedule?	
Monitor session by session; take corrective action if needed.	Summarize at the end of the six-week program (12 sessions).
Are all components of the sessions being provided (e.g., skill building and activity)?	
Monitor session by session; take corrective action if needed.	Complete checklist for at least four of the 12 sessions each semester.
How many young people are participating?	
Take attendance for each session; take corrective action if needed.	Collect attendance for each session; summarize attendance for program.
What do participants like and not like about being in the program?	
Observe/ask participants at each session; take corrective action if needed.	Conduct focus groups at each week of six-week program.
Are program participants having fun?	
Observe/ask participants at each session; take corrective action if needed.	Conduct focus groups at the end of the six-week program.

Data collection methods can be qualitative (descriptive) or quantitative (numeric). Qualitative methods can provide detailed, in-depth information about a specific group. This information, however, might not be representative of the entire target group. Examples of methods that produce qualitative data include in-depth interviews, focus groups, open-ended survey questions, and diaries or logs. In contrast, methods that produce quantitative data involve structured data collection about specific issues and are quantifiable, meaning the data can be summarized using numbers. If proper procedures are followed, they can be representative of the larger target group. Common examples of data collection tools include surveys or questionnaires, record-keeping forms, and direct measures of health indicators such as height and weight (Health Communication Unit, 1997). An overview of some commonly used data collection tools with their strengths and limitations is provided in table 10.5.

Table 10.5 Uses, Strengths, and Limitations
of Various Data Collection Approaches

TOOL AND METHODS	POSSIBLE USES	STRENGTHS AND LIMITATIONS
Record-keeping forms, checklists, other documents Self-completed	• Document activities completed, components included • Document attendance at sessions, events	• Can integrate into normal routine • Fairly easy to design and use • Can provide detailed, accurate information • Can create burden on staff or participants • Might not be completed regularly or accurately
Survey with structured questions and/or scaled responses that can be quantified Written: in person, mailed, Internet Verbal: in person, telephone	• Collect quantifiable information on health behavior, influences on health behavior	• Can collect information from many stakeholders • Can be generalizable • Can minimize interviewer bias • Can collect a lot of information quickly • Requires expertise in selection and design of tool, follow-up procedures, analysis, and interpretation of results • Can be expensive • May lack validity and reliability if tool is poorly designed • Does not provide in-depth view from respondent's perspective
Open-ended survey questions that allow respondent to complete answer in own words Written: mailed, in person, Internet Verbal: in person, telephone	• Add depth to survey results • Explore reasons for answers to close-ended questions • Ask exploratory questions	• Can provide depth • May be time-consuming to analyze • Can add a lot of time for survey completion

(continued)

Table 10.5 *(continued)*

TOOL AND METHODS	POSSIBLE USES	STRENGTHS AND LIMITATIONS
In-depth interviews with semistructured questions Telephone or in person, one-on-one; sometimes audio recorded	• Investigate sensitive issues with a small number of stakeholders • Develop a better understanding of stakeholders' language, opinions, or attitudes	• Involves confidential environment • Limits peer influence • Can explore unanticipated issues that arise in session • Can elicit more detailed information than in focus groups • Requires skilled interviewers • Has potential for interviewer bias • May be more expensive than focus groups • Can be time-consuming to analyze • Results may not be generalizable
Focus group, semistructured discussion with 8-10 stakeholders In person, led by skilled facilitator; usually audio or video recorded	• Gather in-depth information from a small number of stakeholders • Develop a better understanding of stakeholders' language, opinions, or attitudes • Pretest materials with target audience • Develop survey	• Provides in-depth information • Can be easy to implement • Requires skilled facilitators • Requires expertise to design, analyze, and interpret results • Has potential for facilitator bias • Possible influence of participants on one another • May be time-consuming to analyze • Results not generalizable

Adapted from The Health Communication Unit, 1997.

The selection of specific data collection tools and methods depends on a number of factors, starting with the evaluation question. Process evaluation typically uses both quantitative and qualitative approaches. In general, data collection tools such as open-ended interview or focus group questions (qualitative) and written surveys or questionnaires (quantitative) are used to get information from people directly. For observational sources (behavior or environment), a checklist is a commonly used data collection tool. Data sources vary for different evaluation questions and therefore should be identified by question. Examples of data sources, data collection methods, and tools that could be used to evaluate the MMS after-school physical activity program are provided in table 10.6. It is best to use your data collection tools in a small pilot test before using them to collect data for the project.

Use Worksheet 10.3 in the appendix to summarize data sources, data collection methods, and data collection tools for your physical activity program.

Table 10.6 Data Sources, Data Collection Methods, and Data Collection Tools for the MMS After-School Physical Activity Program Process Evaluation Questions

POSSIBLE DATA SOURCES	EXAMPLES OF DATA COLLECTION METHODS AND TOOLS
Is the program being delivered as planned?	
Program leader Observation of program activities	Checklist of desired characteristics of program
Are all sessions being offered on the planned schedule?	
Program leader Sponsoring agency	Schedule of program dates and times, documentation of program activity
Are all components of the sessions being provided (e.g., skill building and activity)?	
Observation of program activities Participants	Checklist of components to be included in program
How many young people are participating?	
Attendance taken by program leader "Head count"	Program attendance list or "head count" for each session
What do participants like and not like about being in the program?	
Program participants	Open-ended questions for participants (written survey or interview, focus group)
Are program participants having fun?	
Observation of participants Participants	Checklist for observation, open-ended questions for participants (written survey or interview, focus groups)

Data Collection Procedures Plan

Data collection procedures describe the specifics of data collection. This includes planning and specifying details of the steps for collecting data on schedule. After the data sources, data collection tools, and data collection methods have been identified and pilot tested, and after timing of data collection has been determined, the following must also be considered:

- A sufficient number of staff are available to collect data.
- Sufficient numbers of data collection tools are available when needed.
- Instructions on how to administer the tools are written down.
- Data collectors are trained to administer the instruments consistently.
- Any permissions or notifications required for collecting data have been obtained.
- Data collectors check completed instruments for missing or invalid information.
- Completed instruments are delivered to the appropriate person(s) for data entry, analysis, and summary.
- Staff roles for the various tasks are clearly defined.

Data Entry, Analysis, and Summary

This part of the plan describes how data will be handled and summarized after they are collected, and how data will be handled if not entered into a computer software program. The plan includes the type of analysis or summary (or both) that will be used to answer the evaluation questions. The goal is to get data into a form that can be summarized and interpreted. Approaches to working with quantitative data are encapsulated in table 9.8. Elements of the plan that deal with qualitative data, including coding of the data, use of data entry and software, and analysis or summary, are provided in table 10.7.

The specific data entry and analysis approach selected is based on the process evaluation question. The following plan illustrates this using the MMS after-school physical activity program.

Table 10.7 Approaches to Coding, Data Entry, and Analysis or Summary for Qualitative Data

PROCESS	EXPLANATION
Examples of data	Written responses to open-ended questions, transcribed interviews and focus group discussions; if transcripts are not feasible, detailed notes are sometimes used.
Coding	Coding involves assigning a word or phrase to similar comments to determine how often the ideas appear in your data.
Software	Some examples of qualitative software: NUD•IST, Ethnograph, NVIVO.
Data entry	After data are coded, software can be used to summarize results. Without software or computer, after data are coded, themes are identified (often by question) and are summarized in bulleted format.
Analysis or summary	Provides a summary of the information collected that is organized to answer evaluation questions.

Adapted from U.S. Department of Health and Human Services, 2002, and The Health Communication Unit, 1997.

Plan for Coding, Data Entry, and Data Analysis or Summary for the MMS After-School Physical Activity Program

Evaluation Question 1

Is the program being delivered as planned?

Coding: Checklist; each desired program characteristic is coded 0 if not checked or 1 if checked.

Data entry/Software: Codes entered into computer by data entry operator.

Data analysis/Summary: Frequencies for each item summed; percent of total items calculated.

Evaluation Question 2

Are all sessions being offered on schedule as planned?

Coding: Checklist; each session is coded 0 if not checked or 1 if checked.

Data entry/Software: Codes entered into computer by data entry operator using Access database.

Data analysis/Summary: Frequencies for each session summed; percent of total sessions calculated.

Evaluation Question 3

Are all components of the sessions being provided (e.g., skill building and activity)?

Coding: Checklist; each component is coded 0 if not checked or 1 if checked.

Data entry/Software: Codes entered into computer by data entry operator using Access database.

Data analysis/Summary: Frequencies for each component summed; percent of total components calculated.

Evaluation Question 4

How many young people are participating?

Coding: Count number of participants at each session.

Data entry/Software: Number at each session entered into Access database.

Data analysis/Summary: Mean number of participants at each session calculated.

Evaluation Question 5

What do participants like and not like about being in the program?

Coding: Themes from focus groups identified and transcripts coded.

Data entry/Software: Codes entered into NUD*IST by data entry operator.

Data analysis/Summary: Summary of themes and issues provided.

Evaluation Question 6

Are program participants having fun?

Coding: Themes identified and written responses to open-ended questions coded.

Data entry/Software: Codes entered into NUD*IST by data entry operator.

Data analysis/Summary: Summary of themes and issues provided.

Use Worksheet 10.4 in the appendix to develop the plan for coding, data entry and software, and data analysis or summary for your program.

Plan for Using Results

It is important to outline your plan for sharing results of the process evaluation with stakeholders, including staff, by answering the following questions:

- How will process monitoring results be shared with staff in a timely manner?
- When and how will summative evaluation results be shared with staff?
- When and how will process evaluation results be shared with program participants and secondary audiences?
- When and how will process evaluation results be shared with other stakeholders, including funding organizations and sponsoring organizations?
- What is the most appropriate channel (e.g., mailing, newsletters, personal contacts, media, Web sites) and format (e.g., summary of methods and results, detailed report with tables and charts, strengths and weaknesses of the program and evaluation, recommendations) for sharing results with each stakeholder group?

Resources Required for Planning and Conducting the Program Evaluation

The next step involves identifying the resources that will be required to plan and carry out the process evaluation. It is important to determine what can be accomplished with existing resources, including staff availability, staff expertise, computers and software, and funding, and what will require seeking outside resources. Options for outside resources include students and faculty from colleges and universities who might be willing to assist with or without financial compensation, personnel from state and local agencies such as health departments, and other consultants or experts who usually work for a fee. The following summary lists resources that may be required for conducting process evaluation. Note that the need for many of the resources listed will depend on the specifics of the individual program.

Summary of Considerations and Resources That May Be Needed for a Process Evaluation Plan

Staff or Consultant Expertise

- For process evaluation and measuring program implementation, quantitative and qualitative data collection methods and analysis
- For coordination of measurement and data-related activities for process evaluation
- For instrument development
- For recruitment and obtaining parent permission
- For data collection
- For data entry and analysis
- For interpreting and reporting results

Materials

- Materials for recruiting participants, including parent information and permission
- Data collection tools (surveys)

Equipment and Supplies

- Equipment for recording and transcription of qualitative data
- Computer equipment and Internet access for records and communication
- Software for data entry and analysis
- Office and other supplies

Facility and Space

- Scheduling and costs
- Space with privacy for data collection

Transportation

Incentives

Other

It is helpful at this point to have a written summary of the process evaluation plan. Use Worksheet 10.5 in the appendix to summarize the overall evaluation plan.

Finally, it is important to develop a detailed work plan that spells out who does what when. These steps ensure that the elements needed for process evaluation are in place and that responsible individuals know what they are supposed to do and when they are supposed to do it. Use Worksheet 10.6 in the appendix to summarize your work plan.

After careful planning and preparation, it is time to carry out your program plan, program effectiveness evaluation plan, and program monitoring (process evaluation) plan! An overview of this process (steps 4-6) is provided next.

Step 4: Carry Out Program and Implement Program Evaluation Plan

In this step, the program plan and the evaluation plan are carried out. Use the program work plan (Worksheet 7.7), the effectiveness evaluation plan (Worksheet 9.6), and the process evaluation plan (Worksheet 10.6) to ensure that all elements of the program and program evaluation are carried out as intended. This step is being taken when the program is "happening"—the planned strategies are being carried out, and program activities are being monitored to ensure that the program is progressing as planned. Of course, planning should minimize problems; however, most programs experience some "growing pains" as they get started. Program implementation often involves problem solving. Some common problems include lower attendance than expected, confusion about roles among those carrying out the program, and unanticipated barriers.

First, identify the problem and its source. Then identify or brainstorm possible solutions, preferably with the help of others on the team, and select the best solution or solutions. Finally, take the steps needed to carry out the solution. What are participation barriers? Is this a transportation issue (children have no way to get home) or a scheduling issue (school day ends too late for program participation)? What will help clarify staff roles? Additional training, routine debriefing, better communication? What is the backup plan if the space for your program is not available on a given day? Make sure that communication about how the program is going is conveyed to program implementers as soon as possible so that needed corrections can be made to keep the program on track in a timely manner.

Step 5: Analyze and Interpret Results

Use Worksheets 9.4 (program effectiveness) and 10.4 (process evaluation) for guidance on coding, data entry, and data analysis. Review evaluation data as they are collected to ensure that there are no problems with the tools used to collect data or the process for gathering and entering data. As already noted, you should ensure that process evaluation results used for program monitoring and early corrective action are available in a timely manner and available to the appropriate program staff. The collection of process and effectiveness data can be an overwhelming task. Staff time must be provided. Efforts to streamline data for easy data entry and analysis may take additional time prior to data collection but will save time once the program has ended. Also, initial data will need to be summarized so that you can interpret your findings. Remember that large volumes of data will need to be collapsed into smaller segments before summarization can occur.

After data have been summarized, evaluate the results while keeping the purpose of the evaluation and the specific evaluation questions in mind (Worksheets 7.3, 9.1, and 10.1). Maintain a focus on the needs and perspectives of the target audience as summaries and reports are developed. Consider the following questions:

- What are the key findings?
- What does the audience for the results need and want to know?
- What are the strengths of the program and its evaluation?
- What are the limitations of the program evaluation (e.g., possible biases, validity and reliability of tools, and generalizability of results)?
- Are there alternative explanations for your results?
- How do your results compare to those of similar programs?
- Are your results consistent with the theory used to develop the program?
- Are your results similar to what you expected? If not, in what ways are they different?

Step 6: Disseminate Results

After the results have been summarized and interpreted, they must be put into a form that can be shared in a timely manner. In this step, previously considered formats and channels of communication with stakeholders are refined. Here are some tips for developing reports, summaries, or recommendations based on evaluation results:

- Consider stakeholders' values; align reports and recommendations with those values when possible.
- Share drafts with stakeholders and solicit feedback from them.
- Remind stakeholders of intended uses of results.
- Relate your reports and recommendations to the original purpose of the evaluation.
- Target reports appropriately for various audiences.
- Summarize key points and issues.
- Keep the language of reports as simple as possible.
- Use charts and tables when appropriate.

SUMMARY

It is important to develop a plan for monitoring your physical activity program to ensure that it is implemented in the way it has been planned and that the intended target audience is reached. The monitoring plan should be based on the details of the program and should include the following components: fidelity, dose delivered, dose received, reach, recruitment, and context. Use the appropriate worksheets developed throughout the planning process to guide you in the implementation phase of the program.

Worksheets

This book focuses on applying theory, developing models, planning evaluation, and integrating evidence from the professional literature to develop programs for children and youth. The process of creating or adapting a physical activity intervention is made easier with the addition of worksheets that facilitate application of the material presented in the book. In the following pages, please find the worksheets referenced throughout the book. These worksheets reflect our interest in developing the capabilities of practitioners to apply theory- and evidence-based approaches to promoting physical activity in children and adolescents. Each worksheet provides a user-friendly guide that assists the reader in developing new programs specific to his or her local area needs and resources. Copy them and use them to help you develop effective physical activity interventions.

APPENDIX

Selecting Theory- and Evidence-Based Approaches to Promote Physical Activity in Children and Youth

STEP	PLANNING FOR YOUR PROGRAM
1. Identify the specific physical activity behavior of interest.	
2. List the most important influences on the physical activity behavior (see tables 2.4 and 2.5 for summary and see other sources).	
a. Individual influences	
b. Interpersonal influences	
c. Organizational influences	
d. Community and environmental influences	
3. Identify intervention methods suggested by theory (see tables 2.6 and 2.7).	
4. Develop specific and practical strategies (see table 2.8 for examples).	

Checklist for Effective Working Teams

____ Obtain representation from all important stakeholders.

____ Develop a common goal or purpose as a group.

____ Define the role of each team member.

____ State the benefits of participation for each team member.

____ Develop a common language and define important terms.

____ Develop a method for effective communication.

____ Develop a meeting schedule that is acceptable to all and considers schedules, workloads, travel distances, parking, and so on.

____ Develop effective team skills: leadership, communication, decision making, and conflict management.

____ Engage in a systematic planning, implementation, and evaluation process.

____ Write down team decisions and plans.

Summary of Progress on Basic Elements

Basic Element 1

Whom is the program designed to serve? How will you gain access to that group?

Basic Element 2

Who can authorize working with the youth, and who will implement the program?

Basic Element 3

Where and when will the program take place, and how will access to that setting be gained?

Basic Element 4

What specific physical activity behaviors will be influenced? (Include intensity, duration, frequency, goal, and type of activity.)

Writing SMART Behavioral Objectives

SMART Objective 1:

Who (priority group):

What behavior (focus of change):

How much (amount of change expected):

When (time frame):

SMART Objective 2:

Who (priority group):

What behavior (focus of change):

How much (amount of change expected):

When (time frame):

Determining Important Influences, Methods, and Program Strategies for Behavioral Objectives

BEHAVIORAL OBJECTIVE	GENERAL METHODS	STRATEGIES AND ACTIVITIES

From *Physical Activity Interventions in Children and Adolescents,* by Dianne S. Ward, Ruth P. Saunders, and Russell R. Pate, 2007, Champaign, IL: Human Kinetics.

Logic Model Template

Inputs	Investments or resources	
Activities	Programs using strategies that target important influences	
Initial effects	Change in important influences	
Intermediate effects	Change in behavior	
Long-term outcomes	Change in health outcomes	

From *Physical Activity Interventions in Children and Adolescents,* by Dianne S. Ward, Ruth P. Saunders, and Russell R. Pate, 2007, Champaign, IL: Human Kinetics.

213

Description and Overview
of Physical Activity Program

1. List stakeholders and describe their role in program planning and implementation:

2. Describe whom program is for and when and where it will take place:

3. State goals and objectives:

4. State the program philosophy or general approach:

5. List and describe the program components or elements, including activity sessions or lessons, as applicable:

6. Describe how change agents will be involved:

7. State the program format and time frame:

Physical Activity Program Work Plan

ACTIVITY	PERSON RESPONSIBLE	COMPLETION DATE
Securing and confirming appropriate space for program activities at the necessary time		
Securing and confirming trained adult leaders to lead program activities (provide training as needed)		
Taking appropriate safety measures for program activities (such as procuring equipment, planning for emergencies)		
Ensuring that participants have safe transportation to and from program		
Promoting program and recruiting participants		
Obtaining appropriate parent or guardian permission or consent		
Ensuring that equipment, materials, and supplies needed to carry out program are available		
Pretesting materials and activities with members of the target audience		
Maintaining communication among program staff and stakeholders		

WORKSHEET 9.1

Program Effectiveness Evaluation Questions

COMPONENT	QUESTION
Behavior change	
Influences on behavior	

Determining Your Evaluation Design
and Sampling Plan
for Program Effectiveness Evaluation

1. How many groups will be evaluated (will the design include a control group)?

2. How will the group(s) be formed?

3. When will evaluation information be collected (will the design include pre- and posttest measures)?

4. What sampling approach will be used to collect information?

5. Describe the final evaluation design:

6. What are the strengths and weaknesses of this design?

Data Sources and Data Collection Tools for Each Effectiveness Evaluation Question

Evaluation Question:

 Data sources:

 Data collection tools:

Evaluation Question:

 Data sources:

 Data collection tools:

Evaluation Question:

 Data sources:

 Data collection tools:

Evaluation Question:

 Data sources:

 Data collection tools:

Planning for Coding, Data Entry/Software, and Data Analysis or Summary

Evaluation Question:

    Coding:

    Data entry/Software:

    Data analysis/Summary:

Evaluation Question:

    Coding:

    Data entry/Software:

    Data analysis/Summary:

Evaluation Question: Coding:

    Data entry/Software:

    Data analysis/Summary:

Summary of Effectiveness Evaluation Plan

ELEMENT	DESCRIPTION
Purposes	
Evaluation questions	
Data sources and sampling	
Data collection tools	
Design	
Data collection procedures	
Data analysis and summary	
Sharing and disseminating results	
Resources needed	

Work Plan for Program Evaluation

TASK	PERSON(S) RESPONSIBLE	COMPLETION DATE
Developing and ensuring linkages to the evaluation plan:		
Evaluation questions (Worksheet 9.1)		
Design and sampling (Worksheet 9.2)		
Measures (Worksheet 9.3)		
Data coding, entry, and analysis (Worksheet 9.4)		
Identifying or developing, then pilot testing evaluation tools		
Collecting data		
Entering and analyzing data		
Interpreting and reporting evaluation results		
Disseminating results		

Process Evaluation Questions and Purposes

COMPONENT	PROCESS EVALUATION QUESTIONS	PURPOSE(S)
Fidelity		
Dose delivered		
Reach		
Dose received		
Recruitment		
Context		

Timing of Data Collection
for Each Process Evaluation Question

Evaluation Question:

   Timing (formative purpose):

   Timing (summative purpose):

Evaluation Question:

   Timing (formative purpose):

   Timing (summative purpose):

Evaluation Question:

   Timing (formative purpose):

   Timing (summative purpose):

Evaluation Question:

   Timing (formative purpose):

   Timing (summative purpose):

Data Sources and Data Collection
Methods and Tools

Evaluation Question:

    Possible data sources:

    Data collection methods and tools:

Evaluation Question:

    Possible data sources:

    Data collection methods and tools:

Evaluation Question:

    Possible data sources:

    Data collection methods and tools:

Evaluation Question:

    Possible data sources:

    Data collection methods and tools:

 From *Physical Activity Interventions in Children and Adolescents,* by Dianne S. Ward, Ruth P. Saunders, and Russell R. Pate, 2007, Champaign, IL: Human Kinetics.

Planning for Coding, Data Entry/Software, and Data Analysis or Summary

Evaluation Question:

Coding:

Data entry/Software:

Data analysis/Summary:

Evaluation Question:

Coding:

Data entry/Software:

Data analysis/Summary:

Evaluation Question:

Coding:

Data entry/Software:

Data analysis/Summary:

Summary of Process Evaluation Plan

ELEMENT	DESCRIPTION
Purposes	
Evaluation questions	
Data sources and sampling	
Data collection tools	
Design	
Data collection procedures	
Data analysis and summary	
Sharing and disseminating results	
Resources needed	

Work Plan for Process Evaluation

TASK	PERSON(S) RESPONSIBLE	COMPLETION DATE
Developing and ensuring linkages to the process evaluation plan:		
Evaluation questions (Worksheet 10.1)		
Timing of data collection (Worksheet 10.2)		
Data sources and tools (Worksheet 10.3)		
Data entry and analysis (Worksheet 10.4)		
Identifying or developing evaluation tools (or both)		
Pilot testing and revising evaluation tools		
Collecting data		
Entering and analyzing data		
Interpreting and reporting evaluation results		
Disseminating results		

From *Physical Activity Interventions in Children and Adolescents,* by Dianne S. Ward, Ruth P. Saunders, and Russell R. Pate, 2007, Champaign, IL: Human Kinetics.

Instruments

The following instruments are referred to throughout the text. Use them to help you develop effective physical activity interventions.

NAP SACC Instrument

Nutrition And Physical Activity Self-Assessment for Child Care

Your Name: _____ Date: _____

Child Care Center/Home Name: _____

Please read each statement or question carefully and check the response that best fits your child care center or home. Your honest responses will help us work with you to build a healthy nutrition and physical activity environment at your center or home.

SECTION I: NUTRITION

(N1) Fruits and Vegetables

A. Fruit (not juice) is served:	☐ 2 times per week or less	☐ 3-4 times per week	☐ 1 time per day	☐ 2 or more times per day
B. Fruit is served fresh, frozen, or canned in own juice:	☐ Rarely or never	☐ Some of the time	☐ Most of the time	☐ All of the time
C. 100% fruit juice is served:	☐ 2 or more times per day	☐ 1 time per day	☐ 2-4 times per week	☐ 1 time per week or less
D. Vegetables (not including french fries or fried potatoes) are served:	☐ 2 times per week or less	☐ 3-4 times per week	☐ 1 time per day	☐ 2 or more times per day
E. Vegetables served are dark green, red, orange, or yellow in color:	☐ Less than 1 time per week	☐ 1-2 times per week	☐ 3-4 times per week	☐ 1 or more times per day
F. Cooked vegetables are prepared with added meat fat, margarine or butter:	☐ 1 or more times per day	☐ 3-4 times per week	☐ 1-2 times per week	☐ Less than 1 time per week

(N2) Fried Foods and High Fat Meats

A. Fried or pre-fried meats (chicken nuggets) or fish (fish sticks) are served:	☐ 1 or more times each day	☐ 3-4 times per week	☐ 1-2 times per week	☐ Less than once a week or never
B. Fried or pre-fried potatoes (french fries, tater tots, hash browns) are served:	☐ 1 or more times each day	☐ 3-4 times per week	☐ 1-2 times per week	☐ Less than once a week or never
C. High fat meats (sausage, bacon, hot dogs, bologna, ground beef) are served:	☐ 1 or more times each day	☐ 3-4 times per week	☐ 1-2 times per week	☐ Less than once a week or never

Ammerman, AS, Benjamin, SE, Sommers, JS, Ward, DS. 2004. The Nutrition and Physical Activity Self-Assessment for Child Care (NAP SACC) environmental self-assessment instrument. Division of Public Health, NC DHHS, Raleigh, NC, and the Center for Health Promotion and Disease Prevention, UNC-Chapel Hill, Chapel Hill, NC.

1

(continued)

D. Lean meats, (baked or broiled chicken, turkey, or fish) are served:	☐ Less than once a week	☐ 1-2 times per week	☐ 3-4 times per week	☐ 1 or more times per day

(N3) Beverages

A. Drinking water is available outside:	☐ Not freely available	☐ Available during designated water breaks	☐ Easily visible and available on request	☐ Easily visible and available for self-serve
B. Drinking water is available inside:	☐ Not freely available	☐ Available during designated water breaks	☐ Easily visible and available on request	☐ Easily visible and available for self-serve
C. Sugary drinks (Kool-aid™, sports drinks, sweet tea, punches, soda) other than 100% juice are served:	☐ 1 or more times each day	☐ 3-4 times per week or never	☐ 1-2 times per week	☐ Less than one time per week
D. Milk served to children ages 2 and older is usually:	☐ Whole or regular	☐ 2% reduced fat	☐ 1% low-fat	☐ Skim or non-fat
E. Soda and other soft-drink vending machines are located:	☐ In entrance or front of building	☐ In public areas but not entrance	☐ Out of sight of parents and children	☐ No vending machines on site

(N4) Menus and Variety

A. Menus used are:	☐ 1-week cycle	☐ 2-week cycle	☐ 3-week or more without seasonal change	☐ 3-week or more with seasonal change
B. Menus include whole grain foods that are high in fiber (whole wheat bread, oatmeal, brown rice, Cheerios™):	☐ 1 time per week or less	☐ 2-4 times per week	☐ 1 time per day	☐ 2 or more times per day
C. Weekly menus include a combination of both new and familiar foods:	☐ Rarely or never	☐ Some of the time	☐ Most of the time	☐ All of the time
D. Weekly menus include foods from a variety of cultures:	☐ Rarely or never	☐ Some of the time	☐ Most of the time	☐ All of the time

(N5) Meals and Snacks

A. When children eat less than half of a meal or snack, the staff help determine if they are full before removing plate:	☐ Rarely or never	☐ Some of the time	☐ Most of the time	☐ All of the time

Ammerman, AS, Benjamin, SE, Sommers, JS, Ward, DS. 2004. The Nutrition and Physical Activity Self-Assessment for Child Care (NAP SACC) environmental self-assessment instrument. Division of Public Health, NC DHHS, Raleigh, NC, and the Center for Health Promotion and Disease Prevention, UNC-Chapel Hill, Chapel Hill, NC.

2

(continued)

B. When children request seconds, staff help children determine if they are still hungry before serving the requested food:	☐ Rarely or never	☐ Some of the time	☐ Most of the time	☐ All of the time
C. Children who are picky eaters (able to eat a food but resisting) are encouraged to try new or less favorite food:	☐ Rarely or never	☐ Some of the time	☐ Most of the time	☐ All of the time
D. Sweets or high fat, high salt foods (cookies, cakes, candy, chips, cheese doodles) are served for snacks:	☐ 1 or more times each day	☐ 3-4 times per week	☐ 1-2 times per week	☐ Less than one time per week
E. Food is used to reward desired behavior:	☐ All of the time	☐ Most of the time	☐ Some of the time	☐ Rarely or never
F. Food is used to control behavior or withheld as punishment:	☐ All of the time	☐ Most of the time	☐ Some of the time	☐ Rarely or never

(N6) Foods Offered Outside of Regular Meals and Snacks

A. Guidelines provided to parents for food brought in for holidays or celebrations are:	☐ Not available	☐ Loose guidelines with healthier options encouraged	☐ Written guidelines for healthier options that are not always enforced	☐ Written guidelines for healthier options that are usually enforced
B. Holidays are celebrated with mostly healthy foods or with non-food treats like stickers:	☐ Rarely or never	☐ Some of the time	☐ Most of the time	☐ All of the time
C. Fundraising consists of selling only non-food items (like wrapping paper, coupon books or magazines):	☐ Rarely or never	☐ Some of the time	☐ Most of the time	☐ All of the time

(N7) Supporting Healthy Eating

A. Children and staff sit down together for meals:	☐ Rarely or never	☐ Some of the time	☐ Most of the time	☐ All of the time
B. Meals are served family style (children serve themselves with limited help):	☐ Rarely or never	☐ Some of the time	☐ Most of the time	☐ All of the time
C. Staff consume the same food and drinks as the children:	☐ Rarely or never	☐ Some of the time	☐ Most of the time	☐ All of the time

Ammerman, AS, Benjamin, SE, Sommers, JS, Ward, DS. 2004. The Nutrition and Physical Activity Self-Assessment for Child Care (NAP SACC) environmental self-assessment instrument. Division of Public Health, NC DHHS, Raleigh, NC, and the Center for Health Promotion and Disease Prevention, UNC-Chapel Hill, Chapel Hill, NC.

3

(continued)

D. Staff eat or drink less healthy foods (especially sweets, salty snacks, and sugary drinks) in front of the children:	☐ All of the time	☐ Most of the time	☐ Some of the time	☐ Rarely or never
E. Staff talk with children about trying and enjoying healthy foods:	☐ Rarely or never	☐ Some of the time	☐ Most of the time	☐ All of the time

(N8) Nutrition Education for Children, Parents, and Staff

A. Training opportunities on nutrition are provided for staff:	☐ Rarely or never	☐ Less than 1 time per year	☐ 1 time per year	☐ 2 times per year or more
B. Nutrition training is provided by qualified professional (nurse, registered dietitian, doctor):	☐ Rarely or never	☐ Some of the time	☐ Most of the time	☐ All of the time
C. Staff provide nutrition education for children:	☐ Rarely or never	☐ 1 time per month	☐ 2-3 times per month	☐ 1 time per week or more
D. Nutrition education opportunities are offered to parents (workshops and activities):	☐ Rarely or never	☐ Less than 1 time per year	☐ 1 time per year	☐ 2 times per year or more

(N9) Nutrition Policy

A. A written policy on nutrition and food service that covers most of the NAP SACC is:	☐ Not available	☐ Available but not followed by most staff	☐ Available but followed only by some staff	☐ Available and routinely followed by all staff

SECTION II: PHYSICAL ACTIVITY

(PA1) Active Play and Inactive Time

A. Active (free) play time is provided to all children:	☐ 15-30 minutes each day	☐ 31-45 minutes each day	☐ 46-60 minutes each day	☐ More than 60 minutes each day
B. Structured physical activity (teacher-led) is provided to all children:	☐ Less than 1 time per month	☐ 2-4 times per month	☐ 2-4 times per week	☐ Daily
C. Outdoor active play is provided for all children:	☐ 1 time per week or less	☐ 2-4 times per week	☐ 1 time per day	☐ 2 or more times per day

Ammerman, AS, Benjamin, SE, Sommers, JS, Ward, DS. 2004. The Nutrition and Physical Activity Self-Assessment for Child Care (NAP SACC) environmental self-assessment instrument. Division of Public Health, NC DHHS, Raleigh, NC, and the Center for Health Promotion and Disease Prevention, UNC-Chapel Hill, Chapel Hill, NC.

4

(continued)

D. Staff restrict active play time for children who misbehave:	☐ Often	☐ Sometimes	☐ Never	☐ Never and provide more active play time to reward
E. Children are seated (excluding nap time) more than 30 minutes at a time:	☐ 1 or more times each day	☐ 3-4 times per week	☐ 1-2 times per week	☐ Less than one time per week or never

(PA2) TV Use and TV Viewing

A. Television use consists of the:	☐ TV turned on most of the day, including meal time, everyday	☐ TV turned on for part of the time, most days	☐ TV turned on everyday for part of the time, some days	☐ TV used rarely and only for viewing educational programs
B. Children are allowed to watch TV, videos or play video games:	☐ Throughout the day	☐ Once a day	☐ 2-4 times per week	☐ 1 time per week or less, usually for educational use only

(PA3) Play Environment

A. Fixed play equipment (swings, slides, climbing equipment, overhead ladders) is:	☐ Unavailable at our site	☐ Swing sets (or one type of equipment) only available	☐ Different equipment available that suits most children	☐ Wide variety of equipment available and accommodates needs of all children
B. Safety checks on equipment occur:	☐ Only when equipment is installed	☐ 1 time per year	☐ 1 time per month	☐ 1 time per week
C. Portable play equipment that stimulates a variety of gross motor skills (wheel toys, balls, tumbling mats) consists of:	☐ Little variety and children must take turns	☐ Some variety but children must take turns	☐ Good variety but children must take turns	☐ Lots of variety for all children to use at the same time
D. When weather is not suitable to go outdoors, indoor play space is available:	☐ For quiet play	☐ For very limited movement (jumping and rolling)	☐ For some active play (jumping, rolling and skipping)	☐ For all activities, including running

(PA4) Supporting Physical Activity

A. During active (free) play time staff:	☐ Rarely or never join children in active play (mostly sit or stand)	☐ Sometimes join children in active play	☐ Often or always join children in active play	☐ Often or always join children in active play and make positive statements about the activity

Ammerman, AS, Benjamin, SE, Sommers, JS, Ward, DS. 2004. The Nutrition and Physical Activity Self-Assessment for Child Care (NAP SACC) environmental self-assessment instrument. Division of Public Health, NC DHHS, Raleigh, NC, and the Center for Health Promotion and Disease Prevention, UNC-Chapel Hill, Chapel Hill, NC.

5

(continued)

B. Staff show visible support for physical activity by:	☐ No posters, pictures, or books about physical activity displayed	☐ A few posters, pictures, or books about physical activity displayed in a few rooms	☐ Posters, pictures, or books about physical activity are displayed in most rooms	☐ Posters, pictures, or books about physical activity are displayed in every room

(PA5) Physical Activity Education for Children, Parents, and Staff

A. Training opportunities are provided for staff in physical activity:	☐ Rarely or never	☐ Less than 1 time per year	☐ 1 time per year	☐ 2 times per year
B. Physical activity training is provided by qualified professional (nurse, athletic trainer, doctor):	☐ Rarely or never	☐ Less than 1 time per year	☐ 1 time per year	☐ 2 times per year
C. Staff provide physical activity education for children:	☐ Rarely or never	☐ 1 time per month	☐ 2-3 times per month	☐ 1 time per week
D. Physical activity education is offered to parents (workshops and activities):	☐ Rarely or never	☐ Less than 1 time per year	☐ 1 time per year	☐ 2 times per year

(PA6) Center Physical Activity Policy

A. A written policy on physical activity that covers most of the NAP SACC areas is:	☐ Not available	☐ Available but not followed by most staff	☐ Available but followed only by some staff	☐ Available and routinely followed by all staff

For more information about this self-assessment instrument and the NAP SACC project, please visit http://www.napsacc.org

Please use the following citation when referencing this instrument: Ammerman, AS, Benjamin, SE, Sommers, JS, Ward, DS. 2004. The Nutrition and Physical Activity Self-Assessment for Child Care (NAP SACC) environmental self-assessment instrument. Division of Public Health, NC DHHS, Raleigh, NC, and the Center for Health Promotion and Disease Prevention, UNC-Chapel Hill, Chapel Hill, NC.

State of North Carolina • Michael F. Easley, Governor | Department of Health and Human Services • Carmen Hooker Odom, Secretary
Division of Public Health • NC Healthy Weight Initiative

Department of Nutrition • UNC Schools of Public Health and Medicine | UNC Center for Health Promotion and Disease Prevention

6

PDPAR Instrument

3 Day Physical Activity Recall (3DPAR)

Instructions:

The purpose of this questionnaire is to approximate the amount of physical activity that you perform. The name of each day (Monday, Sunday, and Saturday) that you will describe is located in the top right hand corner of each time sheet.

1. For **each** time period, write in the activity number that corresponds to the **main** activity you actually performed during that particular time period.

2. Then rate how physically **hard** each activity was. Place a "☞" in the timetable to indicate one of the following intensity levels for each activity.

3. Indicate **where** you performed the activity by writing in the corresponding number.

4. Write the corresponding number for **with whom** you performed the activity in the last column.

Activities Scale:

• **Light** - Slow breathing, little or no movement.

•**Moderate** - Normal breathing and some movement.

• **Hard** - Increased breathing and moderate movement.

• **Very Hard** - Hard breathing and quick movement.

PAR / Version A / January 15, 2002

(continued)

From *Physical Activity Interventions in Children and Adolescents,* by Dianne S. Ward, Ruth P. Saunders, and Russell R. Pate, 2007, Champaign, IL: Human Kinetics.

235

Sample activity time sheet:

The table below shows the correct way to fill out the activity time sheets.
Note that only **one** intensity level is checked for each activity.

	Activity Number	Light	Moderate	Hard	Very Hard	Where	With Whom
7:00-7:30	22	☞				6	0
7:30-8:00	21	☞				6	0
8:00-8:30	18		☞			5	1
8:30-9:00	28	☞				1	3
9:00-9:30	28	☞				1	3
9:30-10:00	26			☞		1	3
10:00-10:30	26			☞		1	3
10:30-11:00	58	☞				1	1

PAR / Version A / January 15, 2002

(continued)

ID _____

MONDAY

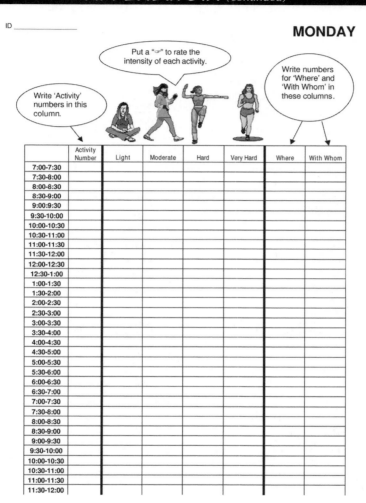

Write 'Activity' numbers in this column.

Put a "☞" to rate the intensity of each activity.

Write numbers for 'Where' and 'With Whom' in these columns.

	Activity Number	Light	Moderate	Hard	Very Hard	Where	With Whom
7:00-7:30							
7:30-8:00							
8:00-8:30							
8:30-9:00							
9:00-9:30							
9:30-10:00							
10:00-10:30							
10:30-11:00							
11:00-11:30							
11:30-12:00							
12:00-12:30							
12:30-1:00							
1:00-1:30							
1:30-2:00							
2:00-2:30							
2:30-3:00							
3:00-3:30							
3:30-4:00							
4:00-4:30							
4:30-5:00							
5:00-5:30							
5:30-6:00							
6:00-6:30							
6:30-7:00							
7:00-7:30							
7:30-8:00							
8:00-8:30							
8:30-9:00							
9:00-9:30							
9:30-10:00							
10:00-10:30							
10:30-11:00							
11:00-11:30							
11:30-12:00							

PAR / Version A / January 15, 2002

(continued)

'Activity' Numbers:

EATING
1. Eating a meal
2. Snacking

WORK
3. Working (e.g., part-time job, child care) (**list**)
_____
4. Doing house chores (e.g., vacuuming, dusting, washing dishes, animal care, etc.)
5. Yard Work (e.g., mowing, raking)

AFTER SCHOOL/SPARE TIME/HOBBIES
6. Church
7. Hanging around
8. Homework
9. Listening to music
10. Marching band/flag line/drill team
11. Music lesson/playing instrument
12. Playing video games/surfing internet
13. Reading
14. Shopping
15. Talking on phone
16. Watching TV or movie

TRANSPORTATION
17. Riding in a car/bus
18. Travel by walking
19. Travel by bicycling

SLEEP/BATHING
20. Getting dressed
21. Getting ready (hair, make-up, etc.)
22. Showering/bathing
23. Sleeping

SCHOOL
24. Club, student activity
25. Lunch/free time/study hall
26. P.E. Class
27. ROTC
28. Sitting in class

PHYSICAL ACTIVITIES
29. Aerobics, jazzercise, water aerobics, taebo
30. Basketball
31. Bicycling, mountain biking
32. Bowling
33. Broomball
34. Calisthenics / Exercises (push-ups, sit-ups, jumping jacks)
35. Canoeing, kayaking
36. Cheerleading, drill team
37. Dance (at home, at a class, in school, at a party, at a place of worship)
38. Exercise machine (cycle, treadmill, stair master, rowing machine)
39. Football
40. Frisbee

41. Golf
42. Gymnastics / Tumbling
43. Hiking
44. Hockey (ice, field, street, or floor)
45. Horseback riding
46. Jumping rope
47. Kick boxing
48. Lacrosse
49. Martial arts (karate, judo, boxing, tai kwan do, tai chi)
50. Playground games (tether ball, four square, dodge ball, kick ball)
51. Playing catch
52. Playing with younger children
53. Roller blading, ice skating, roller skating
54. Riding scooters
55. Running / Jogging
56. Softball / Baseball
57. Skiing (downhill, cross country, or water)
58. Skateboarding
59. Sailing
60. Skimboarding
61. Sledding, tobogganing, bobsledding
62. Snorkeling
63. Snowboarding
64. Snowmobiling
65. Snowshoeing
66. Soccer
67. Surfing (body or board)
68. Swimming (laps)
69. Swimming (play, pool games – Marco Polo, water volleyball)
70. Tennis, racquetball, badminton, paddleball
71. Trampolining
72. Tubing / Rafting
73. Track & field
74. Volleyball
75. Walking for exercise
76. Walking for transportation
77. Weightlifting
78. Wrestling
79. Yoga, stretching
80. Other _____

'Where' Numbers:

1 - SCHOOL GROUNDS
2 - RECREATION CENTER
3 - PARK or PLAYGROUND
4 - GYM
5 - NEIGHBORHOOD
6 - HOME
7 - AT WORK

'With Whom' Numbers:

0 - BY YOURSELF
1 - with 1 OTHER PERSON
2 - with SEVERAL PEOPLE
3 - with a CLASS OR TEA

From *Physical Activity Interventions in Children and Adolescents,* by Dianne S. Ward, Ruth P. Saunders, and Russell R. Pate, 2007, Champaign, IL: Human Kinetics.

SAPAC Instrument

SCHOOL DAY - MONDAY

ACTIVITY	BEFORE SCHOOL			DURING SCHOOL			AFTER SCHOOL		
	# of minutes	With Whom	Where	# of minutes	With Whom	Where	# of minutes	With Whom	Where
PHYSICAL ACTIVITIES									
1. Aerobics, jazzercise, water aerobics, taebo									
2. Basketball									
3. Bicycling, mountain biking									
4. Bowling									
5. Broomball									
6. Calisthenics / Exercises (push-ups, sit-ups, jumping jacks)									
7. Canoeing, kayaking									
8. Cheerleading, drill team									
9. Dance (at home, at a class, in school, at a party, at a place of worship)									
10. Exercise machine (cycle, treadmill, stair master, rowing machine)									
11. Football									
12. Frisbee									
13. Golf									
14. Gymnastics, tumbling									
15. Hiking									
16. Hockey (ice, field, street, or floor)									
17. Horseback riding									
18. Jumping rope									
19. Kick boxing									

PSR / Version A January 15, 2002

Page 1

(continued)

ACTIVITY	BEFORE SCHOOL			DURING SCHOOL			AFTER SCHOOL		
	# of minutes	With Whom	Where	# of minutes	With Whom	Where	# of minutes	With Whom	Where
20. Lacrosse									
21. Martial arts (karate, judo, boxing, tai kwan do, tai chi)									
22. Playground games (tetherball, four square, dodgeball, kickball)									
23. Playing catch									
24. Playing with younger children									
25. Roller blading, ice skating, roller skating									
26. Riding scooters									
27. Running, jogging									
28. Softball / Baseball									
29. Skiing (downhill, cross-country, or water)									
30. Skateboarding									
31. Sailing									
32. Skimboarding									
33. Sledding, tobogganing, bobsledding									
34. Snorkeling									
35. Snowboarding									
36. Snowmobiling									
37. Snowshoeing									
38. Soccer									
39. Surfing (body or board)									
40. Swimming laps									
41. Swimming (play, pool games – Marco Polo, water volleyball)									

PSR / Version A January 15, 2002

(continued)

Page 2

ACTIVITY	BEFORE SCHOOL			DURING SCHOOL			AFTER SCHOOL		
	# of minutes	With Whom	Where	# of minutes	With Whom	Where	# of minutes	With Whom	Where
42. Tennis, racquetball, badminton, paddle ball									
43. Trampolining									
44. Tubing / Rafting									
45. Track & Field									
46. Volleyball									
47. Walking for exercise									
48. Walking for transportation									
49. Weight lifting									
50. Wrestling									
51. Yoga									
52. Other (specify):									
WORK ACTIVITIES									
53. Indoor chores: mopping, vacuuming, sweeping									
54. Outdoor chores: mowing, raking, gardening									
55. Child care									

	BEFORE SCHOOL	AFTER SCHOOL
56. Television or video watching	___ hours plus ___ minutes	___ hours plus ___ minutes
57. Computer/Internet	___ hours plus ___ minutes	___ hours plus ___ minutes
58. Video/Computer games	___ hours plus ___ minutes	___ hours plus ___ minutes
59. Talking on phone	___ hours plus ___ minutes	___ hours plus ___ minutes

PSR / Version A January 15, 2002

Page 3

(continued)

3-DAY SELF-ADMINISTERED PHYSICAL ACTIVITY CHECKLIST (3DSAPAC)
CODING INSTRUCTIONS

PSR / Version A January 15, 2002

MINUTES?

For each activity you did, enter the number of minutes you did the activity during each part of the day – before school, during school, and after school.

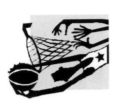

WITH WHOM?

We would like to know **who was with you** when you were doing this activity. Please put:

"0" for activities done BY YOURSELF
"1" if done with 1 OTHER PERSON
"2" for SEVERAL PEOPLE
"3" for WITH A CLASS OR TEAM

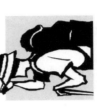

WHERE?

We are also interested in **where you were** while you were doing this activity. Please put:

"1" for SCHOOL GROUNDS
"2" for a RECREATION CENTER
"3" for PARK or PLAYGROUND
"4" for GYM
"5" for NEIGHBORHOOD
"6" for HOME
"7" for AT WORK

QUESTIONS 56-59:

Finally, we are interested in how much time you spent doing each of the activities listed in questions 56-59. Please put the number of hours and minutes you spent doing each of these things, during each part of the day.

Page 10

Self-Efficacy for Physical Activity

Rationale: Self-efficacy is one of the most frequently studied correlates of physical activity (Sallis, Prochaska, & Taylor, 2000). True self-efficacy, often referred to as perceived self-efficacy (Bandura, 1997, p. 3), is defined as "beliefs in one's capabilities to organize and execute the courses of action required to produce given attainments." However, in familiar activities that must be performed regularly to achieve desired results, Bandura suggests that self-regulatory efficacy becomes more salient. This type of efficacy is often operationalized as "barriers efficacy" or the confidence a person has in overcoming barriers to changing his or her behavior. Because of its potential role in moderating the intervention, self-efficacy will be specifically targeted in the intervention, and thus there is a strong rationale for assessing it.

	DISAGREE	NEITHER AGREE NOR DISAGREE	AGREE
1. I can be physically active on most days of the week.			
2. I can ask my parents or other adults to do active things with me.			
3. I can be physically active on most days even if it is very hot or cold outside.			
4. I can do active things because I know how to do them.			
5. I can be physically active even at home.			
6. I can be physically active on most days even if I could watch TV or play video games instead.			
7. I can ask my best friend to be physically active with me on most days.			
8. I have the skill to be active in my free time.			

Adapted from Motl et al., 2000.

Enjoyment of Physical Activity

Objectives:

To measure enjoyment of physical activity for the purposes of (a) determining whether the intervention confers a higher enjoyment of physical activity in the intervention school versus the control school and (b) determining whether enjoyment of physical activity mediates the effects of the intervention.

Methods:

PACES measure (Motl et al., 2001)

WHEN I AM ACTIVE . . .	DISAGREE A LOT	DISAGREE A LITTLE	NEITHER AGREE NOR DISAGREE	AGREE A LITTLE	AGREE A LOT
I feel bored.					
I dislike it.					
it's no fun at all.					
it makes me depressed.					
it frustrates me.					
it's not at all interesting.					
I feel as though I would rather be doing something else.					

Adapted from Motl et al., 2001.

Social Support for Physical Activity

DURING A TYPICAL WEEK, HOW OFTEN . . .	NEVER	SOMETIMES	EVERY DAY
do you encourage your friends to do physical activities or play sports?			
do your friends encourage you to do physical activities or play sports?			
do your friends do physical activities or play sports with you?			
do your friends tell you that you are doing a good job at physical activities or sports?			
has someone encouraged you to do physical activities or play sports?			
has someone done a physical activity or played sports with you?			
has someone provided transportation to a place where you can do physical activities or play sports?			
has someone watched you participate in physical activities or sports?			
has someone told you that you are doing well in physical activities or sports?			

Adapted from Sallis, Taylor, Dowda, Freedson, and Pate 2002.

Aaron, D.J., Kriska, A.M., Dearwater, S.R., Anderson, R.L., Olsen, T.L., Cauley, J.A., & LaPorte, R.E. (1993). The epidemiology of leisure physical activity in an adolescent population. *Medicine and Science in Sports and Exercise,* *25*(7), 847-853.

Allensworth, D.D., & Kolbe, L.J. (1987). The comprehensive school health program: Exploring an expanded concept. *Journal of School Health,* *57*(10), 409-412.

Allensworth, D.D., Lawson, E., Nicholson, L., & Wyche, J. (1997). Building the infrastructure for comprehensive school health programs in grades K-12. In: D.D. Allensworth, E. Lawson, L. Nicholson, & J. Wyche (Eds.), *Schools and health: Our nation's investment* (pp. 237-270). Washington, DC: National Academy Press.

Bandura, A. (1986). *Social foundations of thought and action.* New York: Prentice Hall.

Bandura, A. (1997). *Self-efficacy: The exercise of control.* New York: Freeman.

Baranowski, T., Baranowski, J.C., Cullen, K.W., Thompson, D.I., Nicklas, T., Zakeri, I.F., & Rochon, J. (2003). The Fun, Food and Fitness Project (FFFP): The Baylor GEMS pilot study. *Ethnicity and Disease, 13*(Suppl. 1), 30-39.

Baranowski, T., Hooks, P., Tsong, Y., Cieslik, C., & Nader, P.R. (1987). Aerobic physical activity among third- to sixth-grade children. *Journal of Developmental and Behavioral Pediatrics, 8,* 203-206.

Baranowski, T., & Stables, G. (2000). Process evaluations of the 5-a-day projects. *Health Education and Behavior, 27*(2), 157-166.

Bartholomew, L.K., Parcel, G.S., Kok, G., & Gottlieb, N.H. (2001). *Intervention mapping: Designing theory- and evidence-based health promotion programs.* New York: McGraw-Hill.

Beech, B., Klesges, R.C., Kumanyika, S.K., Murray, D.M., Klesges, L., McClanahan, B., Slawson, D., Nunnally, C., Rochon, J., McLain-Allen, B., & Pree-Cary, J. (2003). Child- and parent-targeted interventions: The Memphis GEMS pilot study. *Ethnicity and Disease, 13*(Suppl. 1), 40-53

Bell, C., & Darnell, J. (1994). Curricular examples of sport education. In D. Siedentop (Ed.), *Sport education.* Champaign, IL: Human Kinetics.

Bricker, S.K., Kanny, D., Mellinger-Birdsong, A., Powell, K.E., & Shisler, J.L. (2002). School transportation modes—Georgia, 2000. *Morbidity and Mortality Weekly Report, 51*(32), 704-705.

Brown, W.H., Pfeiffer, K.A., McIver, K.L., Dowda, M., Almeida, J., & Pate, R.R. (2006). Assessing preschool children's physical activity: The Observational System for Recording Physical Activity in Children—Preschool Version. *Research Quarterly for Exercise and Sport* 77, 167-176.

Caballero, B., Clay, T., Davis, S.M., Ethelbah, B., Holy Rock, B., Lohman, T., Norman, J., Story, M., Stone, E.J., Stephenson, L., & Stevens, J. (2003).

Pathways: A school-based, randomized controlled trial for the prevention of obesity in American Indian schoolchildren. *American Journal of Clinical Nutrition, 78*(5), 1030-1038.

Cavill, N., Biddle, S., & Sallis, J.F. (2001). Health enhancing physical activity for young people: Statement of the United Kingdom Expert Consensus Conference. *Pediatric Exercise Science, 13*(1), 12-25.

Centers for Disease Control and Prevention. (1997). Guidelines for school and community programs to promote lifelong physical activity among young people. *MMWR Recommendations and Reports, 46*(RR-6), 1-36.

Centers for Disease Control and Prevention. (1999). Framework for program evaluation in public health. *MMWR Recommendations and Reports, 48* (No. RR-11) 1-40.

Centers for Disease Control and Prevention. (2000). *CDC growth charts: United States.* Report No. 314. Hyattsville, MD: National Center for Health Statistics.

Centers for Disease Control and Prevention. (2001). Increasing physical activity. A report on recommendations of the Task Force on Community Preventive Services. *MMWR Recommendations and Reports, 50*(RR-18), 1-14.

Centers for Disease Control and Prevention. (2004). Surveillance summaries. *MMWR Recommendations and Reports, 53*(SS-2), 1-96.

Centers for Disease Control and Prevention. (2005). Barriers to children walking to or from school—United States, 2004. *Morbidity and Mortality Weekly Report, 54*(38), 949-952.

Cooper Institute for Aerobics Research. (1999). *FITNESSGRAM test administration manual* (2nd ed.). Champaign, IL: Human Kinetics.

Davison, K.K., Cutting, T.M., & Birch, L.L. (2003). Parents' activity-related parenting practices predict girls' physical activity. *Medicine and Science in Sports and Exercise, 35*(9), 1589-1595.

Dellinger, A.M., & Staunton, C.E. (2002). Barriers to children walking and biking to school—United States, 1999. *Morbidity and Mortality Weekly Report, 51*(32), 701-704.

Dollman, J., Norton, K., & Norton, L. (2005). Evidence for secular trends in children's physical activity behaviour. *British Journal of Sports Medicine, 39,* 892-897.

Doolittle, T.L., & Bigbee, R. (1968). The twelve-minute run-walk: A test of cardiorespiratory fitness of adolescent boys. *Research Quarterly, 39*(3), 491-495.

Dowda, M., Pate, R.R., Trost, S.G., Almeida, M.J.C.A., & Sirard, J. (2004). Influences of preschool policies and practices on children's physical activity. *Journal of Community Health, 29*(3), 183-195.

DuRant, R.H., Baranowski, T., Puhl, J., Rhodes, T., Davis, H., Greaves, K.A., & Thompson, W.O. (1993). Evaluation of the Children's Activity Rating Scale (CARS) in young children. *Medicine and Science in Sports and Exercise, 25*(12), 1415-1421.

Dwyer, T., Coonan, W.E., Leitch, D.R., Hetzel, B.S., & Baghurst, R.A. (1983). An investigation of the effects of daily physical activity on the health of primary school students in South Australia. *International Journal of Epidemiology, 12*(3), 308-313.

Engh, F. (2002). *Why Johnny hates sports.* New York: Square One.

Epstein, L.H. (1998). Integrating theoretical approaches to promote physical activity. *American Journal of Preventive Medicine, 14,* 257-265.

Epstein, L.H., Roemmich, J.N., Paluch, R.A., & Raynor, H.A. (2005). Physical activity as a substitute for sedentary behavior in youth. *Annals of Behavioral Medicine, 29*(3), 200-209.

Ernst, M.P., & Pangrazi, R.P. (1999). Effects of a physical activity program on children's activity levels and attraction to physical activity. *Pediatric Exercise Science, 11,* 393-405.

Evenson, K.R., Hutson, S.L., McMillen, B.J., Bors, P., & Ward, D.S. (2003). Statewide prevalence and correlates of walking and bicycling to school. *Archives of Pediatric and Adolescent Medicine, 157*(9), 887-892.

Faith, M.S., Berman, N., Heo, M., Pietrobelli, A., Gallagher, D., Epstein, L.H., Eiden, M.T., & Allison, D.B. (2001). Effects of contingent television on physical activity and television viewing in obese children. *Pediatrics, 107*(5), 1043-1048.

Federal Interagency Forum on Child and Family Statistics. (2005). America's children: Key national indicators of well-being. Retrieved March 29, 2006, from www.childstats.gov/americaschildren/pop6.asp.

Fetro, J.V. (1998). Implementing coordinated school health programs in local schools. In: E. Marx, S.F. Wooley, & D. Northrop (Eds.), *Health is academic. A guide to coordinated school health programs* (pp. 15-42). New York: Teachers College Press.

Fink, A. (1993). *Evaluation fundamentals. Guiding health programs, research, and policy.* Newbury Park, CA: Sage.

Fitzgibbon, M.L., Stolley, M.R., Dyer, A.R., Van Horn, L., & KauferChristoffel, K. (2002). A community-based obesity prevention program for minority children: Rationale and study design for Hip-Hop to Health Jr. *Preventive Medicine, 34*(2), 289-297.

Fitzgibbon, M.L., Stolley, M.R., Schiffer, L., Van Horn, L., KauferChristoffel, K., & Dyer, A. (2005). Two-year follow-up results for Hip Hop to Health, Jr.: A randomized controlled trial for overweight prevention in preschool minority children. *Journal of Pediatrics, 146*(5), 618-625.

Fogelholm, M., Nuutinen, M., Pasanen, M., Myöhänen, E., & Säätelä, T. (1999). Parent-child relationship of physical activity patterns and obesity. *International Journal of Obesity, 23*(12), 1262-1268.

Ford, B.S., McDonald, T.E., Owens, A.S., & Robinson, T.N. (2002). Primary care interventions to reduce television viewing in African-American children. *American Journal of Preventive Medicine, 22*(2), 106-109.

Fulton, J.E., Garg, M., Galuska, D.A., Rattay, K.T., & Caspersen, C.J. (2004). Public health and clinical recommendations for physical activity and physical fitness: Special focus on overweight youth. *Sports Medicine, 34*(9), 581-599.

Gittelsohn, J., Steckler, A., Johnson, C.C., Pratt, C., Grieser, M., Pickrel, J., Stone, E.J., Conway, T., Coombs, D., & Staten, L.K. (2006). Formative research in school and community-based health programs and studies: "State of the art" and the TAAG approach. *Health Education and Behavior, 33*(1), 25-39.

Glanz, K., Rimer, B.K., & Lewis, F.M. (2002). Theory, research, and practice in health behavior and health education. In: K. Glanz, B.K. Rimer, & F.M. Lewis (Eds.), *Health behavior and health education: Theory, research, and practice* (3rd ed., pp. 22-39). San Francisco: Jossey-Bass.

Goldfield, G.S., Kalakanis, L.E., Ernst, M.M., & Epstein, L.H. (2000). Open-loop feedback to increase physical activity in obese children. *International Journal of Obesity, 24*(7), 888-892.

Gordon-Larsen, P., Griffiths, P., Bentley, M.E., Ward, D.S., Kelsey, K., Shields, K., & Ammerman, A. (2004). Barriers to physical activity: Qualitative data on caregiver-daughter perceptions and practices. *American Journal of Preventive Medicine, 27*(3), 218-223.

Gordon-Larsen, P., McMurray, R.G., & Popkin, B.M. (2000). Determinants of adolescent physical activity and inactivity patterns. *Pediatrics, 105*(6), E83-90.

Gordon-Larsen, P., Nelson, M.C., Page, P., & Popkin, B.M. (2006). Inequality in the built environment underlies key health disparities in physical activity and obesity. *Pediatrics, 117*(2), 417-424.

Gortmaker, S.L., Chueng, L.W., Peterson, K.E., Chomitz, G., Cradle, J.H., Dart, H., Fox, M.K., Bullock, R.B., Sobol, A.M., Colditz, G., Field, A.E., & Laird, N. (1999). Impact of a school-based interdisciplinary intervention on diet and physical activity among urban primary school children: Eat Well and Keep Moving. *Archives of Pediatric and Adolescent Medicine, 153*(9), 975-983.

Gortmaker, S.L., Peterson, K., Wiecha, J., Sobol, A.M., Dixit, S., Fox, M.K., & Laird, N. (1999). Reducing obesity via a school-based interdisciplinary intervention among youth: Planet Health. *Archives of Pediatric and Adolescent Medicine, 153*(4), 409-418.

Green, L.W., & Kreuter, M.W. (1999). *Health promotion planning: An educational and environmental approach* (3rd ed.). Mountain View, CA: Mayfield.

Gustafson, S.L., & Rhodes, R.E. (2006). Parental correlates of physical activity in children and adolescents. *Sports Medicine, 36*(1), 79-97.

Harrell, J.S., McMurray, R.G., Bangdiwala, S.I., Frauman, A.C., Gansky, S.A., & Bradley, C.B. (1996). The effects of a school-based intervention to reduce cardiovascular risk factors in elementary school children: The Cardiovascular Health in Children (CHIC) Study. *Journal of Pediatrics, 128*(6), 797-804.

Hastie, P.A. (1998). Skill and tactical development during sport education season. *Research Quarterly for Exercise and Sport, 69*(4), 368-379.

Health Communication Unit. (1997). *Evaluating health promotion programs.* Toronto: Centre for Health Promotion, University of Toronto.

Heitzler, C.D., Martin, S.L., Duke, J., & Huhman, M. (2006). Correlates of physical activity in a national sample of children aged 9-13 years. *Preventive Medicine, 42*(4), 254-260.

Hoefer, W.R., McKenzie, T.L., Sallis, J.F., Marshall, S.J., & Conway, T.L. (2001). Parental provision of transportation for adolescent physical activity. *American Journal of Preventive Medicine, 21*(1), 48-51.

Jackson, A.S., & Coleman, A.E. (1976). Validation of distance run tests for elementary school children. *Research Quarterly, 47*(1), 86-94.

Kahn, E.B., Ramsey, L.T., Brownson, R.C., Heath, G.W., Howze, E.H., Powell, K.E., Stone, E.J., Rajab, M.W., Corso, P., & Task Force on Community Preventive Services. (2002). The effectiveness of interventions to increase physical activity: A systematic review. *American Journal of Preventive Medicine, 22*(4S1), 73-107.

Kann, L., Warren, C.W., Harris, W.A., Collins, J.L., Douglas, K.A., Collins, M.E., Williams, B.I., Ross, J.G., & Kolbe, L.J. (1995). Youth risk behavior surveillance—United States, 1993. *Morbidity and Mortality Weekly Report, 44*(1), 1-56.

Kelder, S., Hoelscher, D.M., Barroso, C.S., Walker, J.L., Cribb, P., & Hu, S. (2005). The CATCH Kids Club: A pilot after-school study for improving elementary students' nutrition and physical activity. *Public Health Nutrition, 8*(2), 133-140.

Kohl, H.W. III, & Hobbs, K.E. (1998). Development of physical activity behaviors among children and adolescents. *Pediatrics, 101*(3, Pt. 2), 549-554.

Liu, N.Y., Plowman, S.A., & Looney, M.A. (1992). The reliability and validity of the 20-meter shuttle test in American students 12 to 15 years old. *Research Quarterly for Exercise and Sport, 63*(4), 360-365.

Lowry, R., Wechsler, H., Kann, L., & Collins, J.L. (2001). Recent trends in participation in physical education among US high school students. *Journal of School Health, 71*(4), 145-152.

Luepker, R.V., Perry, C.L., McKinlay, S.M., Nader, P.R., Parcel, G.S., Stone, E.J., Webber, L.S., Elder, J.P., Feldman, H.A., & Johnson, C.C. (1996). Outcomes of a field trial to improve children's dietary patterns and physical activity: The Child and Adolescent Trial for Cardiovascular Health. *Journal of the American Medical Association, 275*(10), 768-776.

Maksud, M.G., & Coutts, K.G. (1971). Application of the Cooper twelve-minute run-walk test to young males. *Research Quarterly, 42*(1), 54-59.

Manios, Y., Kafatos, A., & Markakis, G. (1998). Physical activity of 6-year-old children: Validation of two proxy reports. *Pediatric Exercise Science, 10*(2), 176-188.

McKenzie, T.L., Cohen, D.A., Sehgal, A., Williamson, S., & Golinelli, D. (2006). System for observing play and recreation in communities (SOPARC): Reliability and feasibility measures. *Journal of Physical Activity and Health, 3*(Suppl. 1), S208-222.

McKenzie, T.L., Marshall, S.J., Sallis, J.F., & Conway, T.L. (2000). Leisure-time physical activity in school environments: An observational study using SOPLAY. *Preventive Medicine, 30*(1), 70-77.

McKenzie, T.L., Marshall, S.J., Sallis, J.F., & Conway, T.L. (2000). Student activity levels, lesson context and teacher behavior during middle school physical education. *Research Quarterly for Exercise and Sport, 71*(3), 249-259.

McKenzie, T.L., Nader, P.R., Strikmiller, P.K., Yang, M., Stone, E.J., Perry, C.L., Taylor, W.C., Epping, J.N., Feldman, H.A., Luepker, R.V., & Kelder, S.H. (1996). School physical education: Effect of the Child and Adolescent Trial for Cardiovascular Health. *Preventive Medicine, 25*(4), 423-431.

McKenzie, T.L., Sallis, J.F., & Nader, P.R. (1991). SOFIT: System for observing fitness instruction time. *Journal of Teaching Physical Education, 11,* 195-205.

McKenzie, T.L., Sallis, J.F., Patterson, T., Elder, J.P., Berry, C.C., Rupp, J.W., Atkins, C.J., Buono, M.J., & Nader, P.R. (1991). BEACHES: An observational system for assessing children's eating and physical activity behaviors and associated events. *Journal of Applied Behavior Analysis, 24*(1), 141-151.

McKenzie, R.L., Sallis, J.F., Prochaska, J.J., Conway, T.L., Marshall, S.J., & Rosengard, P. (2004). Evaluation of a two-year middle school physical education intervention: M-SPAN. *Medicine and Science in Sports and Exercise, 36*(8), 1382-1388.

McKenzie, T.L., Stone, E.J., Feldon, H.A., Epping, J.N., Yang, M., Strikmiller, P., Lytle, L.A., & Parcel, G.S. (2001). Effects of the CATCH physical education instruction: Teacher type and lesson location. *American Journal of Preventive Medicine, 21*(2), 101-109.

McLeroy, K.R., Bibeau, D., Steckler, A., & Glanz, K. (1988). An ecological perspective on health promotion programs. *Health Education Quarterly, 15*(4), 351-377.

Metz, K.F., & Alexander, J.F. (1970). An investigation of the relationship between maximum aerobic work capacity and physical fitness in twelve- to fifteen-year-old boys. *Research Quarterly, 41*(1), 75-81.

Minkler, M., & Wallerstein, N.B. (2002). Improving health through community organization and community building. In: K. Glanz, B.K. Rimer, & F.M. Lewis (Eds.), *Health behavior and health education: Theory, research, and practice* (3rd ed.). New York: Wiley.

Mischel, W. (1973). Toward a cognitive social learning reconceptualization of personality. *Psychological Review, 80*(4), 252-283.

Morgan, D.W., Tseh, W., Caputo, J.L., Keefer, D.J., Craig, I.S., Griffith, K.B., Akins, M., Griffith, G.E., Krahenbuhl, G.S., & Martin, P.E. (2002). Prediction of the aerobic demand of walking in children. *Medicine and Science in Sports and Exercise, 34*(12), 2097-2102.

Motl, R.W., Dishman, R.K., Saunders, R., Dowda, M., Felton, G., & Pate, R.R. (2001). Measuring enjoyment of physical activity in adolescent girls. *American Journal of Preventive Medicine, 21*(2), 110-117.

Motl, R.W., Dishman, R.K., Trost, S.G., Saunders, R.P., Dowda, M., Felton, G., Ward, D.S., & Pate, R.R. (2000). Factorial validity and invariance of questionnaires measuring social-cognitive determinants of physical activity among adolescent girls. *Preventive Medicine, 31*(5), 584-594.

Murphy, J.K., Alpert, B.S., Christman, J.V., & Willey, E.S. (1988). Physical fitness in children: A survey method based on parental report. *American Journal of Public Health, 78*(6), 708-710.

Myers, L., Strikmiller, P.K., Webber, L.S., & Berenson, G.S. (1996). Physical and sedentary activity in school children grades 5-8: The Bogalusa Heart Study. *Medicine and Science in Sports and Exercise, 28,* 852-859.

Nader, P.R. (2003). Frequency and intensity of activity of third grade children in physical education. *Archives of Pediatric and Adolescent Medicine, 157*(2), 185-190.

National Association for Sport and Physical Education (NASPE). (1995). *Moving into the future: National standards for physical education. A guide to content and assessment.* Boston: McGraw-Hill. Portions available at www.aahperd. org/naspe/.

National Center for Chronic Disease Prevention and Health Promotion. (2004). BMI for children and teens. Atlanta, GA: Centers for Disease Control and Prevention. Retrieved September 29, 2006, from http://www.cdc.gov/nccd-php/dnpa/bmi/bmi-for-age.htm.

National Center for Health Statistics. (2004). Prevalence of overweight among children and adolescents: United States, 1999-2000. Retrieved September 29, 2006, from www.cdc.gov/nchs/products/pubs/pubd/hestats/overwght99. htm.

National Institute of Child Health and Human Development Study of Early Child Care and Youth Development. (2003). Frequency and intensity of activity of third-grade children in physical education. *Archives of Pediatric and Adolescent Medicine, 157*(2), 185-190.

Neumark-Sztainer, D., Story, M., Hannan, P., & Rex, J. (2003). New Moves: A school-based obesity prevention program for adolescent girls. *Preventive Medicine, 37*(1), 41-51.

Noland, M., Danner, F., DeWalt, K., McFadden, M., & Kotchen, J.M. (1990). The measurement of physical activity in young children. *Research Quarterly for Exercise and Sport, 61*(2), 146-153.

Nutrition and Physical Activity Work Group. (2002). *Guidelines for a comprehensive program to promote healthy eating and physical activity.* Champaign, IL: Human Kinetics.

Parcel, G.S., Simons-Morton, B., O'Hara, N.M., Baranowski, T., & Wilson, B. (1989). School promotion of healthful diet and physical activity: Impact on learning outcomes and self-reported behavior. *Health Education Quarterly, 16*(2), 181-199.

Pate, R.R. (1988). The evolving definition of fitness. *Quest, 40*(3), 174-179.

Pate, R.R., Pratt, M., Blair, S.N., Haskell, W.L., Macera, C.A., Bouchard, C., Buchner, D., Ettinger, W., Heath, G.W., & King, A.C. (1995). Physical activity and public health. A recommendation from the Centers for Disease Control and Prevention and the American College of Sports Medicine. *Journal of the American Medical Association, 273*(5), 402-407.

Pate, R.R., Ross, R., Dowda, M., Trost, S.G., & Sirard, J. (2003). Validation of a three-day physical activity recall instrument in female youth. *Pediatric Exercise Science, 15*(3), 257-265.

Pate, R.R., & Sirard, J.S. (2000). Physical activity in young people. *Topics in Nutrition, 8*(1), 1-18.

Pate, R.R., Trost, S.G., Mullis, R., Sallis, J.F., Wechsler, H., & Brown, D.R. (2000). Community interventions to promote proper nutrition and physical activity among youth. *Preventive Medicine, 31*(Suppl. 1), 138-149.

Pate, R.R., Ward, D.S., Saunders, R.P., Felton, G., Dishman, R.K., & Dowda, M. (2005). Promotion of physical activity among high-school girls: A randomized controlled trial. *American Journal of Public Health, 95*(9), 1582-1587.

Patrick, K., Calfas, K.J., Norman, G.J., Zabinski, M.F., Sallis, J.F., Rupp, J., Covin, J., & Cella, J. (2006). Randomized controlled trial of a primary care and home-based intervention for physical activity and nutrition behaviors. *Archives of Pediatric Adolescent Medicine, 160,* 128-136.

Patrick, K., Sallis, J.F., Lydston, D., Prochaska, J.J., Calfas, K.J., Zabinski, M., Wilfley, D., & Saelens, B. (2001). Preliminary evaluation of a multi-component program for nutrition and physical activity change in primary care: PACE+ for adolescents. Archives *of Pediatrics and Adolescent Medicine, 155*(8), 940-946.

Perry, C.L., Sellers, D.E., Johnson, C., Pedersen, S., Bachman, K.J., Parcel, G.S., Stone, E.J., Luepker, R.V., Wu, M., Nader, P.R., & Cook, K. (1997). The Child and Adolescent Trial for Cardiovascular Health (CATCH): Intervention, implementation, and feasibility for elementary schools in the United States. *Health Education and Behavior, 24*(6), 716-735.

Plescia, M., Young, S., & Ritzman, R.L. (2005). Statewide Community-based Health Promotion: A North Carolina Model to Build Local Capacity for Chronic Disease Prevention. *Preventing Chronic Disease: Public Health Research, Practice and Policy.* Vol 2. Special Issue: November 2005. Retrieved September 29, 2006, from http://www.cdc.gov/pcd/issues/2005/nov/pdf/05_0058.pdf.

Prochaska, J.J., Zabinski, M.F., Calfas, K.J., Sallis, J.F., & Patrick, K. (2000). PACE+: Interactive communication technology for behavior change in clinical settings. *American Journal of Preventive Medicine, 19*(2), 127-131.

Puhl, J., Greaves, K., Hoyt, M., & Baranowski, T. (1990). Children's Activity Rating Scale (CARS): Description and calibration. *Research Quarterly for Exercise and Sport, 61*(1), 26-36.

Pucher, J., & Dijkstra, L. (2003). Making walking and cycling safer: Lessons from the Netherlands and Germany. *American Journal of Public Health, 93*(9), 1509-1516.

Ransdell, L.B., Detling, N., Hildebrand, K., Lau, P., Moyer-Mileur, L., & Shultz, B. (2005). Daughters and Mothers Exercising Together (DAMET): Effects of home- and university-based physical activity interventions on perceived benefits and barriers related to exercise. *American Journal of Health Studies, 19*(5), 195-204.

Ransdell, L.B., Detling, N., Taylor, A., Reel, J., & Shultz, B. (2004). Daughters and Mothers Exercising Together (DAMET): Effects of home- and university-based physical activity interventions on physical self-perception. *Women and Health, 39*(2), 63-82.

Ransdell, L.B., Taylor, A., Oakland, D., Schmidt, J., Moyer-Mileur, L., & Shultz, B. (2003). Daughters and Mothers Exercising Together: Effects of home- and community-based programs. *Medicine and Science in Sports and Exercise, 35*(2), 286-296.

Rekers, G.A., Sanders, J.A., Strauss, C.C., Rasbury, W.C., & Morey, S.M. (1989). Differentiation of adolescent activity participation. *Journal of Genetic Psychology, 150*(3), 323-335.

Resnicow, K., Yaroch, A.L., Davis, A., Wang, D.T., Carter, S., Slaughter, L., Coleman, D., & Baranowski, T. (2000). GO GIRLS!: Results from a nutrition and physical activity program for low-income, overweight African American adolescent females. *Health Education and Behavior, 27*(5), 616-631.

Roberts, D.R., Foehr, U.G., & Rideout, V. (2005). *Generation M: Media in the lives of 8-18 year-olds.* Menlo Park, CA: Kaiser Family Foundation. Retrieved September 29, 2006, from www.kff.org/entmedia/entmedia030905pkg.cfm.

Roberts, D.F., Foehr, U.G., Rideout, V.J., & Brodie, M. (1999). *Kids & media @ the new millennium.* Menlo Park, CA: Kaiser Family Foundation. Retrieved September 29, 2006, from www.kff.org/entmedia/1535-index.cfm.

Robinson, R.N. (1999). Reducing children's television viewing to prevent obesity. *Journal of the American Medical Association, 282*(16), 1561-1567.

Robinson, T.N., Kraemer, H.C., Matheson, D.M., Pruitt, L.A., Owens, A.S., Flint-Moore, N.M., Davis, G.J., Emig, K.A., Brown, R.T., Rochon, J., Green, S., & Varady, A. (2003). Dance and reducing television watching to prevent weight gain in African American girls: Stanford GEMS pilot study. *Ethnicity and Disease, 13*(Suppl. 1), 65-77.

Rubenstein, H., Sternbach, M.R., & Pollack, S.H. (1999). Protecting the health and safety of working teenagers. *American Family Physician, 60*, 575-587.

Safrit, M.J. (1973). *Evaluation in physical education. Assessing motor behavior.* Englewood Cliffs, NJ: Prentice Hall.

Sallis, J., Alcaraz, J., McKenzie, T., Hovell, M., Kolody, B., & Nader, P. (1992). Parental behavior in relation to physical activity and fitness in 9-year-old children. *American Journal of Diseases of Children, 146*, 1383-1388.

Sallis, J.F., Buono, M.J., Roby, J., Micale, F.G., & Nelson, J.A. (1993). Seven-day recall and other physical activity self-reports in children and adolescents. *Medicine and Science in Sports and Exercise, 25*(1), 99-108.

Sallis, J.F., & Glanz, K. (2006). The role of built environments in physical activity, eating, and obesity in childhood. *Future Child, 16*(1), 89-108.

Sallis, J.F., McKenzie, T.L., Alcaraz, J.E., Kolody, B., Faucette, N., & Howell, M.F. (1997). Effects of a 2-year health-related physical education program (SPARK) on physical activity and fitness in elementary school students. Sports, Play, and Active Recreation for Kids. *American Journal of Public Health, 87*(8), 1328-1334.

Sallis, J.F., McKenzie, T.L., Conway, T.L., Elder, J.P., Prochaska, J.J., Brown, M., Zive, M.M., Marshall, S.J., & Alcaraz, J.E. (2003). Environmental interventions for eating and physical activity: A randomized controlled trial in middle schools. *American Journal of Preventive Medicine, 24*(3), 209-217.

Sallis, J.F., McKenzie, T.L., Kolody, B., & Curtis, P. (1996). Assessing district administrators' perceptions of elementary school physical education. *Journal of Physical Education, Recreation and Dance, 67*(8), 25-29.

Sallis, J.F., & Owen, N. (2002). Ecological models of health behavior. In: K. Glanz, B.K. Rimer, & F.M. Lewis (Eds.), *Health behavior and health education: Theory, research, and practice* (3rd ed., pp. 462-484). San Francisco: Jossey-Bass.

Sallis, J.F., & Patrick, K. (1994). Physical activity guidelines for adolescents: Consensus statement. *Pediatric Exercise Science, 302*(6), 314.

Sallis, J.F., Pinski, R.B., Grossman, R.M., Patterson, T.L., & Nader, P.R. (1988). The development of self-efficacy scales for health-related diet and exercise behaviors. *Health Education Research, 3*(3), 283-292.

Sallis, J.F., Prochaska, J.J., & Taylor, W.C. (2000). A review of correlates of physical activity of children and adolescents. *Medicine and Science in Sports and Exercise, 32*(5), 963-975.

Sallis, J.F., & Saelens, B.E. (2000). Assessment of physical activity by self-report. Status, limitations, and future directions. *Research Quarterly for Exercise and Sport, 71*(Suppl. 2), S1-14.

Sallis, J.F., Strikmiller, P.K., Harsha, D.W., Feldman, H.A., Ehlinger, S., Stone, E.J., Williston, J., & Woods, S. (1996). Validation of interviewer- and self-administered physical activity checklists for fifth grade students. *Medicine and Science in Sports and Exercise, 28*(7), 840-851.

Sallis, J.F., Taylor, W.C., Dowda, M., Freedson, P.S., & Pate, R.R. (2002). Correlates of vigorous physical activity for children in grades 1 through 12: Comparing parent-reported and objectively measured physical activity. *Pediatric Exercise Science, 14*(1), 30-44.

Sammann, P. (1998). *Active youth: Ideas for implementing CDC physical activity promotion guidelines.* Champaign IL: Human Kinetics.

Saunders, R.P., Evans, M.H., & Joshi, P. (2005). Developing a process evaluation plan for assessing health promotion program implementation: A how-to guide. *Health Promotion Practice* 6, 134-147.

Shadish, W.R., Cook, T.D., & Campbell, D.T. (2002). *Experimental and quasi-experimental designs for generalized causal inference.* Boston: Houghton Mifflin.

Siedentop, D. (1994). *Sport education: Quality PE through positive sport experiences.* Champaign, IL: Human Kinetics.

Siedentop, D., Hastie, P.A., & Vander Mars, H. (2002). *Complete guide to sport education.* Champaign, IL: Human Kinetics.

Sindelar, R. (2002). The Clearinghouse on Early Education and Parenting (CEEP). Recess: Is it needed in the 21st century? Retrieved March 29, 2006, from http://ceep.crc.uiuc.edu/poptopics/recess.html.

Sirard, J.R., Ainsworth, B.E., McIver, K.L., & Pate, R.R. (2005). Prevalence of active commuting at urban and suburban elementary schools in Columbia, SC. *American Journal of Public Health, 95*(2), 236-237.

Sirard, J., & Pate, R.R. (2001). Physical activity assessment in children and adolescents. *Sports Medicine, 31*(6), 439-454.

Steckler, A., & Linnan, L., Eds. (2002). *Process evaluation for public health interventions and research.* San Francisco: Jossey-Bass.

Stevens, J., Murray, D.M., Catellier, D.J., Hannon, P.J., Lytle, L.A., Elder, J.P., Young, D.R., Simons-Morton, D.G., & Webber, L.S. (2005). Design of the Trial of Activity in Adolescent Girls. *Contemporary Clinical Trials, 26*(2), 223-233.

Stewart, J.A., Dennison, D.A., Kohl, H.W. III, & Doyle, J.A. (2004). Exercise level and energy expenditure in the Take 10! in-class physical activity program. *Journal of School Health, 74*(10), 397-400.

Stolley, M.R., & Fitzgibbon, M.L. (1997). Effects of an obesity prevention program on the eating behavior of African American mothers and daughters. *Health Education and Behavior, 24*(2), 152-164.

Stone, E.J., McKenzie, T.L., Welk, G.J., & Booth, M.L. (1998). Effects of physical activity interventions in youth: Review and synthesis. *American Journal of Preventive Medicine, 15*(4), 298-315.

Story, M., Kaphingst, K.M., & French, S. (2006). The role of child care settings in obesity prevention. *Future Child, 16*(1), 43-68.

Story, M., Sherwood, N.E., Himes, J.H., Davis, M., Jacobs, D.R., Cartwright, Y., Smyth, M., & Rochon, J. (2003). An after school obesity prevention program for African American Girls: The Minnesota GEMS pilot study. *Ethnicity and Disease, 13*(Suppl. 1), 54-64.

Stratton, R.K. (1996, November/December). Maintaining a positive team environment. Coaching Youth Sports, 2. Retrieved September 29, 2006, from https://courseware.vt.edu/users/rstratto/CYS/.

Strong, W.B., Malina, R.M., Blimkie, C.J., Daniels, S.R., Dishman, R.K., Gutin, B., Hergenroeder, A.C., Must, A., Nixon, P.A., Pivarnik, J.M., Rowland, T., Trost, S., & Trudeau, F. (2005). Evidence based physical activity for school-age youth. *Journal of Pediatrics, 146*(6), 719-720.

Sturm, R. (2005). Childhood obesity—what we can learn from existing data on societal trends, part 1. *Preventing Chronic Disease, 2*(1).

Taggart, A.C., Taggart, J., & Siedentop, D. (1986). Effects of a home-based activity program. A study with low fitness elementary school children. *Behavior Modification, 10*(4), 487-507.

Trost, S., Kerr, L., Ward, D.S., & Pate, R.R. (2001). Physical activity and determinants of physical activity in obese and non-obese children. *International Journal of Obesity, 25*(6), 822-829.

Trost, S.G., Pate, R.R., Sallis, J.F., Freedson, P.S., Taylor, W.C., Dowda, M., & Sirard, J. (2002). Age and gender differences in objectively measured physical activity in youth. *Medicine and Science in Sports and Exercise, 34*(2), 350-355.

Trost, S.G., Sirard, J.R., Dowda, M., Pfeiffer, K.A., & Pate, R.R. (2003). Physical activity in overweight and non-overweight preschool children. *International Journal of Obesity, 27*(7), 834-839.

Tudor-Locke, C., & Bassett, D.R., Jr. (2004). How many steps/day are enough? Preliminary pedometer indices for public health. *Sports Medicine, 34*(1), 1-8.

Tudor-Locke, C., Pangrazi, R.P., Corbin, C.B., Rutherford, W.J., Vincent, S.D., Raustorp, A., Tomson, L.M., & Cuddihy, T.F. (2004). BMI-referenced standards for recommended pedometer-determined steps/day in children. *Preventive Medicine, 38*(6), 857-864.

Tudor-Locke, C., Williams, J.E., Reis, J.P., & Pluto, D. (2002). Utility of pedometers for assessing physical activity: Convergent validity. *Sports Medicine, 32*(12), 795-808.

U.S. Department of Education. (2005). Contexts of elementary and secondary education. Institute of Educational Science. National Center for Educational Statistics. Retrieved March 29, 2006, from http://nces.ed.gov/programs/coe/2005/section4/table.asp?tableID=283.

U.S. Department of Health and Human Services. (1996). *Physical activity and health: A report of the Surgeon General.* Atlanta: Centers for Disease Control and Prevention, National Center for Chronic Disease Prevention and Health Promotion.

U.S. Department of Health and Human Services. (2000). *Healthy people 2010* (2nd ed.). Washington, DC: U.S. Government Printing Office. Retrieved September 29, 2006, from www.healthypeople.gov.

U.S. Department of Health and Human Services. (2002). *Physical activity evaluation handbook.* Atlanta: Centers for Disease Control and Prevention. Retrieved September 29, 2006, from www.cdc.gov/nccdphp/dnpa/physical/handbook/.

U.S. Department of Health and Human Services. (2004). Participation in high school physical education—United States, 1991-2003. *Mortality and Morbidity Weekly Report, 53*(36), 844-847.

U.S. Department of Health and Human Services, & U.S. Department of Education. (2000). Promoting better health for young people through physical activity and sports. Silver Spring, MD: Centers for Disease Control and Prevention. Retrieved September 29, 2006, from www.cdc.gov/HealthyYouth/physicalactivity/promoting_health/index.htm.

Ward, D.S., Evenson, K.R., Vaughn, A., Rodgers, A.B., & Troiano, R.P. (2005). Accelerometer use in physical activity: Best practices and research recommendations. *Medicine and Science in Sports and Exercise, 37*(11), S582-S588.

Welk, G.J. (1999a). Promoting physical activity in children: Parental influences. Washington, DC: ERIC Clearinghouse on Teaching and Teacher Education (ERIC Digest EDO-SP-1999-1). Retrieved September 29, 2006, from www.ericdigests.org/2000-3/activity.htm.

Welk, G.J. (1999b). The youth physical activity promotion model: A conceptual bridge between theory and practice. *Quest, 51*(1), 5-23.

Welk, G.J., Wood, K., & Morss, G. (2003). Parental influences on physical activity in children: An exploration of potential mechanisms. *Pediatric Exercise Science, 15*(1), 19-33.

Weston, A.T., Petosa, R., & Pate, R.R. (1997). Validity of an instrument for measurement of physical activity in youth. *Medicine and Science in Sports and Exercise, 29*(1), 138-143.

Wetzstein, C. (2000, April 13). Latchkey children statistics unlocked. *Washington Times.* Retrieved March 19, 2006, from National Center for Policy Analysis Web site: www.ncpa.org/pi/edu/pd041300c.html.

Wiley, J.F., & Shaver, L.G. (1972). Prediction of maximum oxygen intake from running performances of untrained young men. *Research Quarterly, 43*(1), 89-93.

Young, D.R., Johnson, C.C., Steckler, A., Gittelsohn, J., Saunders, R.P., Saksvig, B.I., Ribisl, K.M., Lytle, L.A., & McKenzie, T.L. (2006). Data to action: Using formative research to develop intervention programs to increase physical activity in adolescent girls. *Health Education and Behavior, 33*(1), 97-111.

Youth Risk Behavior Surveillance System. (2004). Youth online—comprehensive results. Centers for Disease Control and Prevention. Retrieved September 29, 2006, from http://apps.nccd.cdc.gov/yrbss/.

Note: The italicized *f* and *t* following page numbers refer to figures and tables, respectively.

Dianne Stanton Ward, EdD, is a professor and director of the Intervention and Policy Division in the department of nutrition at the University of North Carolina at Chapel Hill. Dr. Ward has more than 30 years' experience in the development and evaluation of physical activity programs for children and adolescents. She has received 10 years of National Institutes of Health (NIH) funding for intervention research and is a member of the NIH Study Section on Community Influences on Health Behavior, a Health of the Public Integrated Review Group.

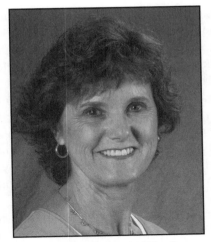

Dianne Stanton Ward

Dr. Ward has received several awards, including the Distinguished Alumni Award in 2001 from the College of Health and Human Performance at the University of North Carolina at Greensboro. She is a fellow in the American College of Sports Medicine, and she is a member of the American Public Health Association, the Association for Nutrition Science, the North American Association for the Study of Obesity, the American Alliance for Health, Physical Education, Recreation and Dance (AAH-PERD), and the North American Society for Pediatric Exercise Medicine. In her leisure time she enjoys hiking, playing golf and tennis, reading, and gardening.

Ruth P. Saunders, PhD, is an associate professor in the department of health promotion, education, and behavior in the Arnold School of Public Health at the University of South Carolina at Columbia. Dr. Saunders has

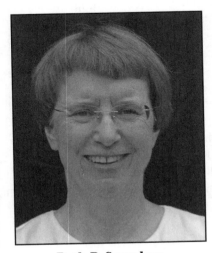

Ruth P. Saunders

worked with physical activity interventions for children and adolescents for more than 10 years and has taught health behavior theory and health promotion program planning and evaluation for 20 years. She has also worked with schools and school districts on health and wellness issues for 18 years.

Dr. Saunders was on the team that developed the Centers for Disease Control and Prevention guidelines for promoting physical activity in school and community settings and has been an active member of a successful research team in obtaining funding and publishing in the area of child and adolescent physical activity and interventions. She has also been an effective collaborator with community organizations and agencies, including schools.

Dr. Saunders has won teaching and research awards and is a member of the American School Health Association, AAHPERD, the Society for Public Health Education, and the American College of Sports Medicine. She enjoys jogging, cycling, gardening, and baking in her spare time.

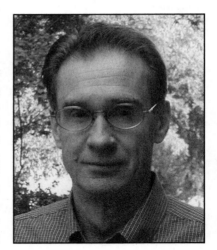

Russell R. Pate, PhD, is a professor in the department of exercise science in the Arnold School of Public Health at the University of South Carolina at Columbia. Dr. Pate has 30 years of experience in researching the issues involved in physical activity interventions. In that time he has received 15 years of NIH funding for research in physical activity interventions. He has also served on the IOM panel for Preventing Childhood Obesity as well as the U.S. Dietary Guidelines Committee. In addition, Dr. Pate has served as

Russell R. Pate

president of the American College of Sports medicine and the National Coalition for Promoting Physical Activity. Dr Pate is a lifelong distance runner. He enjoys traveling and reading.

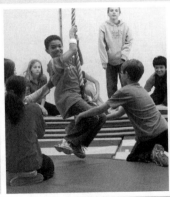
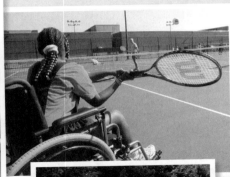
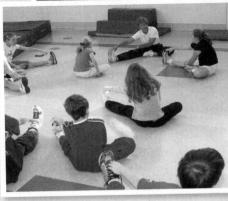
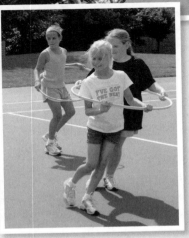

You'll find other outstanding
physical education resources at
www.HumanKinetics.com